A Vow Called Tenderness:

A Path of Spirituality and Sexuality in Friendship and Marriage

A Vow Called Tenderness:

A Path of Spirituality and Sexuality in Friendship and Marriage

By

Maria A. T. Maier

ISBN 1-58500-687-4

About the Book

While many have written about the problems and difficulties in dualism, this book courageously attempts a solution. Beginning with the historical conflicts within psychology by Freud and others of sexual behavior and feminine experience, the author brings the reader to an understanding that sex as we know it is purely a social construct. With this in mind, even the "facts of life" in terms of goal-oriented penetration (with subsequent fears of pregnancy and disease) is no longer a given, or even considered to be more natural.

The response is a revolution in love that begins with the ecstatic experience of mystical union on its ability to offer direct, unmitigated truth. Out of this very real and physical pleasure we are invited to work from the inside out, and unravel many of the myths and painful struggles with which our current understanding of sexuality is fraught. In groundbreaking detail, concrete articulations of an experience of highest consciousness that the mystics themselves did not discuss is brought to the reader. And solid, attainable, duplicatable results for the average self-reflective person are documented along with a step by step formula.

The result is a liberation that provides new postures and deeper intimacy in loving and lovemaking with neither the dangers of disease and immorality of a Liberal model nor the return to rigidity of staid Conservatism and old sexual roles and mores. Because feminine issues are at the core of any sexual construct, women will find a freedom in the untangling of common social assumptions which might cause a woman's sexuality (no longer a liability) to make sense for the very first time.

Maria A.T Maier
A Vow Called Tenderness

Table of Contents

Introduction

The question I am asked most frequently is "what led you to write about the topic of mystical spirituality and sexuality?" Each and every time the answer would be different. This was not because of any shift on my part, though my intellectual and psychological understanding necessarily has evolved considerably over years of research and experience. But rather, it was due to the audience at hand, and whatever aspect of my tender research seemed to present itself most prominently at that moment. Gradually, I found that there seemed to be something in this pile of words, struggles and ecstasies that resonated with everyone on some level. Indeed, it is to further this resonance that is the purpose of writing this book. It is, and I pray I am faithful to, about that which is intrinsic to being human at its core.

The stories poured out, only after I began to articulate something that was not sexually incriminating for women; and for men, the reverse. Men needed to know that this could be explicitly naked, and not something they could only have with a hug. One woman related a story about a yoga spirituality retreat where in one of the exercises she had her arms about a friend for an extended period of time. Her friend was pregnant, and the intimacy stayed on her mind for a very long time. It was an experience that seemed to cause her best sexual experiences to pale in comparison.

To a male companion, I suggested the scenario of being naked with another person and surrendering into that person for no sexual gain or orgasm. He became very moved, as he remembered a personal experience and noticed "I have only had a glimpse of that, a couple of times in my life. But only a glimpse." Long after he was still affected by our discussion of this type of experience and went on to share it with friends.

Sometimes the stories came from the stage, as in the case of one woman who shared a very full and intimate life including what was to her a happy marriage, two very healthy children and intimate friendships. Then she expressed her surprise when after becoming involved in a spiritual direction relationship with a celibate religious nun, "I did not think it possible that two people could be so close."

Often it is an unexpected touch, longer than usual, that brings forth the memory that lasts a lifetime. What if we could create the space for such powerful intimacy, bringing it into our lives as the rule rather than the exception?

To do that, we would have to carefully undo the wrappings of our cultural reality that seems to have such a love consciousness firmly trapped inside. We also require a special lens with which to apprehend and identify exactly what this consciousness and experience is, apart from its imitators. Then, we could offer to liberate it. It would be a trinity of purpose; but also an overwhelming task.

I can only hope to begin the work of possibly pointing to what a myriad of works on dualism have been trying to uncover for many years. The lens I will apply is that of mystical spirituality, which is only too suitable because of its claim of direct, unmitigated insight and revelation. Mysticism, as a work that thrives on the consciousness of love, can shine most clearly on moments that create milestones on our soul's journey.

The liberation of this powerful form of intimacy begins here. It is realized in good women and men of strong consciousness who mandated that this book be written. I am reminded of a wonderful quote attributed to Sufi Hasan of Basra who believed, "where hope is greater than fear, the heart rots". (The type of fear that is referred to here is not a phobia, but rather the kind that is afraid of breaking something that is precious.) The heart of God, which holds the consciousness of this enormous love creates an awesome responsibility and urgency, and a great fear indeed.

Out of this fear, I pursue an articulation and liberation of a rich form of intimacy. May it give glory to the beautiful hearts, bodies and souls of human kind, and to God within us all.

Sex Myths

Studies in the area of developmental psychology indicate how profound our need for human touch is. Harry Harlow in his classic research with rhesus monkeys showed how very young monkeys are behaviorally more aggressive and unable to mate successfully when they have been nurtured by a prefabricated mother made of wire netting.[i] There are reports of higher intelligence among children who are raised in affectionate home environments and numerous other findings relating to the efficacy of massage and the spiritual and physical healing of touch.

Often these findings are placed within a clinical or therapeutic context. Or, as in matters of tender intimacy, this is often placed within the category of sexual maturity and erotic or romantic love. But the purpose of this study is to uncover a form of nongenital lovemaking that is so powerful it is able to stand alone and define itself apart from any current understanding of sexual behavior. The tender encounter most closely resembles the act of sex, in the common perception of the mutual inclination that sexual desire motivates; therefore in order to differentiate between the two, we must explore the physical boundaries and intentionalities of various forms of touch. Most importantly, we must articulate what is and what isn't sexual behavior; and what forms of touch are and which are not motivated by sexual urges or instincts.

Although there are some attempts being made to determine the effects of sexual activity on psychosexual maturity, unlike forms of nonsexual touch, there is no evidence that we as humans are found lacking in any way if we refrain from genital sexual participation. In spite of many contemporary rejections of Freud's notion of a singular sex instinct, our culture retains old associations between sexual desires and sexual needs. Sex, however is not just like eating. Noone ever became emaciated from lack of sex. There is now new evidence that persons who live without a sexual partner are not more sexually frustrated or more prone to masturbation as a form of release.[ii] In fact, the reverse is true. Persons who are sexually active generally engage in more sexual behaviors of all kinds. Instead of having a sexual appetite satiated, sexual activity seems to beget more, not less "hunger".

The time honored linkages between dreams, fantasies and the real desires of patients in psychoanalysis is another area that is being refuted by sex researchers and sociologists, especially those who are concerned about women's sexual identity. Rape and other fantasies by women are not seen as having any connection with a real desire to be forcibly penetrated or even emotionally subjugated by a man. *Sexual Contradictions* is the apt title of a scholarly work by Janet Sayers who echoes throughout the book her own response and challenge to numerous psychoanalytic theories on sex differences. "if - as Gilligan, Keller, Benjamin and Chodorow claim - women do not experience themselves as independent agents in social interaction then where does women's assertion, not least these authors' assertion of their independence and autonomy, come from?"[iii]

Making any judgements of health, normal behavior and what is real desire for a person or a group or a whole sex has its problems, especially when these conclusions are drawn from the context of a different (masculine) sexual perspective and lack substantive behavioral and physiological evidence. This has been a chronic pitfall of the Psychological Sciences. As recently as 1966, Masters and Johnson made the crucial discovery that the female may experience orgasm in only one way, clitorally, debunking the Freudian myth[iv] that mature orgasm for a woman could only occur vaginally. Though this seemed to set some women free of sexual pressures and stereotypes, women continued to be treated as dysfunctional if they could not regularly enjoy orgasm with their partners, with various treatment programs recommended as a "cure".[v]

Finally, the surprising responses from *The Hite Report* and the famous Ann Landers survey demonstrated that women would just as soon cuddle as have sex, that it is physical affection, and not the drive for orgasm women most often feel in need of, and can't seem to get enough of. This new awareness is most often touted as being unique to women, and no special reconstruction of psychological theory has yet been associated with it. The full ramifications of this knowledge, however, carry with it the burden of reevaluating many of our sexual assumptions, notably that sex (the drive) is the primary mover of our affections. And if this is true for women, it may also give us clues as to the deeper affectional needs of men that may be signaled by and not necessarily satisfied by their urges for genital intercourse.

Some like Carl Jung have parted with Freud by maintaining that there is more to the sex instinct than sexual satisfaction. There is primarily a need for intimate or connective union according to Jung although sexual desire is very much a part of this libidinous instinct. Basically an energy of desire, it becomes transformed into any activity, and can be seen as the longing for a sexual other and the longing for union with God.[vi] "Desire does not want pleasurable discharge only"[vii] but also a deeper integration, a joining of polarities, the anima and animus which is at the center of desire.[viii]

There is a clear problem with a theory of polarities in today's age where homosexual desire is recognized as having the same properties, including the "falling in love" experience as heterosexual desire. We have no conclusive evidence of the source of homosexual behavior or even what defines homosexuality. It has even become general knowledge that we are all bisexual to some degree. To chase after and declare polarities in all of our love relationships is suspiciously like finding differences between two human beings. These are certain to exist, but their discovery is not profound or enlightening. Also, a theory of sexual instinct, with a meeting of primitive needs at its base, that can then be transmuted into higher forms of libido, also ignores feminine sexual experience which places a premium on non-genital physical intimacy. Or, it must then assume that most women are naturally born into a higher state of being. The last difficulty with Jung's theory of eros is that it permanently cements love's longings with sexual desire.

Is sex really "making love"? Is all love sexual? Masters and

Johnson comment, "Some moralists would be happier if it could be proven that sex without love does not work. There is no evidence, however, that sex is always or usually better if you are in love. We have worked with hundreds of loving, committed relationships where the sexual interaction was in a shambles and with hundreds of people who deeply enjoyed sex without being in love."[ix] Moreover, sex between two persons who love one another can be lacking in interpersonal and sensitive communication, have a character of being hurried and mechanical, and the sexual intercourse of two persons who hardly know one another can be sublime in its capacity to demonstrate the subtleties of eros and slow, tender love.

The challenge of addressing some of these questions has also been taken on by a contemporary moral philosopher, Roger Scruton who in his work emphasizes the unitive aspect of sexual desire and the subsequent lessening of these desires in a committed sexual relationship until one comes to be "at home" in the arms of a spouse. For Scruton, union is the real aim of desire and orgasm is a distraction from, and ultimately a failure in the achievement of this aim. He quotes Sartre that, "'the full pressing together of the flesh of two people against one another is the true goal of desire' ... I however do not want to press against your flesh for the sake of whatever comfortable sensation this may provide, but for the sake of the consciousness with which your flesh is saturated." In my caresses, Sartre argues, I 'incarnate' you: that is, I summon your consciousness (your 'for-itself') into your flesh, so as to be able to possess you there."[x]

This description of erotic behavior is valuable, because it seems to separate out the involuntary behavior that can be 'summoned', from other forms of physical closeness and affection that leave the participants totally free and voluntary in their response. Also useful is Sartre's claim that the pressing together of two bodies, and not necessarily the goal of orgasm is the real aim of desire. This would seem to more inclusively approximate a sexual theory that is reflective of feminine as well as masculine experience.

But Scruton adds the involuntary or aroused dimension of sexual behavior as a necessary component in the aim of desire.

4

"The aim of desire is first to incarnate the first-person perspective (the for-itself) of the other; and secondly to unite with it as flesh."[xi]

Scruton neglects totally any dialogue of an alternate feminine dimension in viewing sexuality, in spite of wide spread acknowledgement of this at the time of his published work. Finally, his conclusion of whether or not sexual desire is also love, smacks of the traditional view that "men use love to get sex": "Desire does not imply love; but it provides a motive to love - and this fact is crucial in understanding the intentionality of desire. 'Falling in love' is not to be seen as a transition from the absence of love to the presence of love, but rather as the sudden acquisition of this motive."[xii]

A feminine response might be that love provides a motive for desire. The common phrase that "women use sex to get love" might place Scruton's assumptions in a "chicken or the egg" battle of which comes first.

There are other issues that Scruton does not resolve satisfactorily. He does not explain how it is that we love our children in an embodied way, and suggests that we do not as parents have sexual feelings toward our children. This ignores some maternal nursing experiences, and the sexual feelings many fathers have toward their daughters. He does not include religious experience with any attempt to explain what is a very physical yet nongenitally focussed mystical encounter with God or what is often an attendant disappearance of overall sexual tension or desire by its participants. He also does not discuss sexual desire for other persons once his version of "at home-ness" with the spouse is achieved. The happy ending associated with his theory also implies that sexual desire is finally satisfied in the "happy" marriage. This is simply a myth, as explained earlier. Having a partner may bring more sexual desire and tension into one's life, and not the implied abatement or relief from frustration that single or celibate persons are presumed to be in need of.

So the field of philosophy has not improved upon the domain of psychology, primarily because they both choose a limited discourse that stays within select areas of knowledge.

What is really needed is a theory of sexual behavior that can roam into each of the sciences and shed some light instead of the persistent confusion we are offered surrounding our sexuality. This is a serious concern in our current climate of sexual irresponsibility. Robert Moore, Jungian analyst is pointed in his criticism: "Psychoanalysts of all schools tend to avoid the application of insights from the sociology of religion to their practice of psychoanalysis. In this arena, however, the abysmal ignorance of many psychotherapists and psychoanalysts in anthropology and sociology has clinical and ethical implications that must not be ignored. Our lack of attention to perspectives provided by the sociology of knowledge, cultural anthropology, and ethnopsychiatry keeps us from seeing our myopic cultic assumptions and behaviors."[xiii]

It would seem at least that there is room for thought and dissent within prevalent theories of psychology, and some questions and even possible theories might be derived from a feminine awareness and the traditions of religious knowledge. I would like to turn to some of these now and explore some wisdom that these sources of understanding have to offer our conventional concepts of sexuality.

A FEMININE SEXUALITY

God created man in the image of himself, in the image of God he created him, male and female he created them. (Genesis 1: 27)

Like an icon we somehow are reflective of the Divine, and like any icon, the fullness of its message becomes transmuted and pertinent into the present and transcends any other age and all diversity of culture. Our patriarchal tradition has never dialogued about the actual embodied nature of the first humans, preferring a more pure and spiritual cognizance. Somehow the body and nature came to be associated with our uncontrollable and sinful selves, a formidable lifelong opponent that we are condemned to battle and bend to our higher, more spiritual and God given intentions. With or without what has popularly become known as "dualism," it is fruitful to examine what the bodies of Adam and Eve communicate to us about the blueprint of God even before their Fall from Grace.

There are differing thoughts about what the first transgression was. One notion is that Adam and Eve had sexual intercourse for the first time. We are naturally led to wonder what they were doing with one another before the Fall. If not sex, then what? And some may really wonder how any other option could be paradise at all. A glimpse at anatomy is curious, since the first male was created with breasts. Why breasts? There is nothing on the female form that is as conspicuously extraneous. Yet the man was created first, it is written. We can make a game of guessing that God intended to create woman all along, or even that perhaps God created Woman first, since she contains more of the essential configurations and Man looks much more like he was added on to. But does this have anything to say about the image we are created in? Do breasts and the nurturing and reassuring symbols we associate with them have anything to offer our vision of our Creator?

There is also the stigma which our society has handed down through history that since woman came to help man, therefore God all along intended for woman to be an imperfect subordinate, though useful for man's purposes, an inferior being by her very nature. Indeed, the flipside of this could be that God felt that man needed help, and was deficient in his inability to be alone, and besides, we don't find God in scripture sending bad help where there is a need. Typically, God will send an angel, prophet, Paraclete, Jesus, or some other exceptional creature in order to get a job done. In this case, if God created woman because He felt that "it is not good for man to be alone" it is much more consistent to think that He formed a loneliness 'expert' out of Adam's rib.

Indeed, the helping professions are overflowing with literature on male and female differences, much of which is dialogue on how more often than not, it is a woman that a man will look toward to fill his intimacy needs, and a woman similarly, will look toward a woman to fill her needs for intimate relationship. A video series on relationships by Gary Smalley opens with the key that "...Women seem to come equipped with a built-in marriage manual. And if a man learns to tap into it - their relationship can begin to blossom and grow as a result...".[xiv] Men more often will entertain unrealistic expectations of instant intimacy within a relationship,[xv] and their nurture or nature based aggressive and competitive behavior does not easily lend itself to fostering intimacy. Though men are certainly capable of intimacy, Masters and Johnson speculate, "Perhaps the real dilemma of the sex-differences-in-intimacy problem has been aptly described by Rubenstein and Shaver in their 1982 book, *In Search of Intimacy,* who point out that although 'men and women need intimacy to the same degree... fewer women than men get their needs met, despite women's expertise, because so many men are intimacy takers rather than givers.'"[xvi]

Non-genital physical intimacy is a prime area where many women feel shortchanged, and where sexual aggressiveness seems to win any competition or dialogue. In an interesting fashion, sex may be a prime place where men can be takers of non-genital physical intimacy, because the way of traditional sexual intercourse brings only one-third of all women to orgasm on a regular basis. Yet an acceptance of standard sexual pronouncements that all physical intimacy has a genitally based instinct places urges first and women, who simply want to cuddle, last. The short sexual fuse that is common to the male and therefore to our society may be placing all of our relationships out of focus. Because demonstrations of physical affection are most often held in check out of fear that our touch will be misconstrued as sexual, it is important that we attempt to ferret out what is an instinct or a need for physical affection and intimacy that is simply for itself and whether or not it must necessarily be centered in the drive for orgasm.

We must acknowledge that our body is filled with organs that contain many functions and which respond not only to organic stimuli but also to the many emotions that we may be filled with or moved by on any given day. Without much time spent here, I began to think of the tears and the stomach as just a couple of examples. A case of gastric distress could be caused by eating the wrong thing, not having eaten in a long while, or by stress of some sort. "Butterflies" at the beginning of a presentation or performance. We would never, however, develop an instinct of eating as satisfying somehow the "butterflies" phenomenon, or suggest that it is somehow based in the stomach. Tears also have a biological and an emotional function, though we would never suggest a need to cry to be at the base of all of our sorrow. As far as raw emotion is concerned, anger for example, we have numerous options of physical expression. But we don't link any of these with a physical inclination or instinct, such as to kill. The direct association of an emotion such as anger with an expression of physical violence would deeply inhibit most of us from making any verbal admission of anger. It might constrict our actions and even playful taps or smacks; and could also overload our imaginations with thoughts of anger that we dare not naturally express.

So our behavior in kind can become predetermined when we read what popular author Scott Peck writes in his bestseller *The Road Less Traveled:*

When a person falls in love what he or she certainly feels is 'I love him' or 'I love her'. But two problems are immediately apparent. The first is that the experience of falling in love is specifically a sex-linked erotic experience. We do not fall in love with our children even though we may love them very deeply. We do not fall in love with our friends of the same sex - unless we are homosexually oriented - even though we may care for them greatly. We fall in love only when we are consciously or unconsciously sexually motivated.[xvii]

In discussions and workshops, there have been many interesting reactions to Peck's declaration. Initially, many are disbelieving that such an assumption exists in our psychological culture, but once I read the above quote, quickly accept and assert it as fact. There are many problems with the statement that falling in love is motivated by a desire to genitally join to another.

There are first some ironies. Psychotherapy is rooted in the belief that healing is brought about often by the release of feelings that were once repressed out of guilt or the lack of acceptance or credence of others. Central to any healing profession is that the doctor must not attempt to guide or direct the symptoms of the patient, but rather be a sounding board, trusting the truth of the experience as related by the patient. The implication, that irrespective of what a person says, and what their feelings are, they are told they have a certain motivation ipso facto their experience, begets a new version of repression and guilt. This dynamic of reverse repression has been an unfortunate downside to psychotherapy throughout its history and has imprisoned the feminine gender in particular.

It is also ironic that it is specifically those persons who are in love that are most offended by the implication that their feelings are based in selfish or genital urges. There are many questions and confusions as well. During the onslaught of an infatuation, the root word of which means "false fire", it can seem maddening to try to discern whether or not the love felt is genuine or merely lust. And then once a relationship is genitalized, its quality is changed. If sex is invariably at the root of our love encounters, one wonders that sex doesn't deepen or fully satisfy our relationships instead of altering them.

We also need to question how, in the cultural understanding that Peck reflects, an individual can fall in love with God. This is a genuine experience, and mystics have been psychoanalyzed as having overt sexual cravings. But our current understanding of higher consciousness acknowledges that there is a difference between the mystical encounter and having something like sex with God. Indeed, as we will notice in later chapters, recognition of the spirituality of another person seems to affect much in the way of desire and attraction between persons.

Our love for our children may be a powerful example of love that can contain sexual feelings yet be separate from a falling in love encounter. Fathers have confessed struggles with sexual feelings toward their daughters and we know that nursing can illicit sexual stirrings. Why we don't fall in love with our children does more to counter Peck's argument than substantiate it.

Many thoughts, feelings and even other body parts, such as the breasts stimulate our sexual organs. Nursing mothers are keenly aware of a tender and pleasurable function that may stir some genital feelings but is certainly not urgently centered in that part of the body, and not originating in that part of the body. We have ample reason to believe that there are many other feelings that may stir or trigger genital responses of some sort but these do not necessarily indict us to our subconscious desires or even our conscious fantasies. Stress, depression, traumas of all kinds, can increase the urgency of our genital functioning or erase it altogether. On the positive end, we know that a little bit of wine, but not too much enhances lovemaking. A walk in the park, meditation techniques, exercise can add to the whole impact of our sexual performance.

It is not unreasonable to propose that there is another instinct which is at the root of our love relationships, and one that is characterized by a longing for tender closeness. Its instinct might be that of nurture, feeding, protection and surrender. It would be breast and bowels centered (though misperception or a short sexual fuse may not see it so clearly). But mothers and some fathers, most women and some men, know that it is a different way to love, that is not goal oriented or possessive, but is unconditional and liberating.

But is there real evidence that something nongenital though very physically intimate is at the root of our love relationships? And can we demonstrate that it is more satisfying than genitally centered activity? I believe that we are right now experiencing the seeds of a revolution in this regard, and the first place that we can evidence any new movements is in the field of the marriage therapy professions.

TENDER INSTINCTS

Many marriage manuals are now advocating and encouraging nongenital touch as a way to enhance intimacy and love within a relationship. Some of this has come about as a way of meeting feminine needs, as Gary Smalley notes, "the average woman needs from 8 to 10 meaningful touches from a loved one each day to remain physically and emotionally healthy."[xviii] He goes on to assert that men could add years to their life if they responded in kind. Another area of awareness has come from therapy techniques for sexual dysfunction, especially the ground breaking method that Masters and Johnson first developed, which involve several stages of a 'sensate focus' program where touch without the goal of sex brings remarkable cures.

The most recent Chicago survey of male and female human sexual behavior indicate that not much has changed from other surveys that show how only one third of all women orgasm regularly from intercourse. Though I already mentioned that this may be an interesting place where many males actually receive nongenital and 'instant intimacy' from women who are not able to respond sexually in intercourse, it is valuable to notice that women in spite of this still prefer traditional postures of intercourse to other forms of sexual congress.

An early published work by Marriage Encounter suggests that there are four ways a partner can respond emotionally to the other partner whose sexual needs may be greater than their own. That partner is usually the woman, and of the range of possibilities - duty, resentment, psychological rape - the last is what the authors' refer to as a deeper, "maternal joy in giving life. There is a very close bond between the marriage bed and the delivery table in more ways than one...Where a woman has this freedom to be herself in making love, and where there is an other-centered love to express, a difference in sexual appetite isn't an insoluble problem. Sexual intercourse can be enjoyed and lived on many different levels. Some women even report that they are *most deeply moved* when the erotic element is absent."[xix](Italics mine)

Later in life, a couple who are past childbearing years may enjoy a heightened expression of sexuality because the urgent athleticism of goal centered sex has faded. This is sometimes attributed to changes in the male sexual response. "As a man gets older he takes longer to climax and there are times when he is satisfied without ejaculation. This makes him a better lover."[xx]

This phenomenon of nonsexual sex is not one that falls easily within the predominant male range of sexual experience, but is what brings us back to our original topic, that there are deeply involving nonsexual experiences that cause our erotic or goal centered experiences to pale in comparison. Sex researcher

Paul Pearsall in his book *Super Marital Sex* discovers a similar response in his clients who for medical reasons might not be able to enjoy the biological peak of orgasm. In spite of their physical limitations, these individuals described an emotionally and physically ecstatic type of enjoyment during the act of sex with their partner. Pearsall coined the term "Psyche-asm" and developed a new form of sexual interaction that has 'psychasm' and not orgasm as its goal. Pearsall describes this new form of sex as transpersonal, involving the spiritual, emotional and physical union of two persons. He also advances further the understanding that the less goal (or orgasm) centered sex becomes, the better, the more "super" the sex overall.

In what is a growing movement rapidly becoming mainstream, the demand for something more to connect a couple during our times of high divorce and fast paced lives has driven the rediscovery of Eastern Tantric forms of sexual intercourse. Those like Charles and Caroline Muir and Margo Anand have adapted for the West ways of interaction for couples that increase and deepen the emotion and spirituality between them. It is not, in the words of Charles Muir, a way to make sex better. Rather, it is a way to add meaning and conscious loving into a couple's physical relationship.

The question remains, what if we remove orgasm entirely? Though it is extremely rare, there are celibate married couples who describe themselves as "extremely affectionate" but who do not push one another to the point of arousal or orgasm. Gabrielle Brown in her book *The New Celibacy* interviews three such married couples. The individuals had some similar characteristics. They all seem to have had considerable sexual experience in earlier years that they thoroughly enjoyed. The age range was thirty to fifty. Before trying celibacy they also had the supportive friendship of other celibate couples they knew and cited this as an important element. Most importantly, negative religious or spiritual reasons were not mentioned for their celibacy, but rather the desire for a deeper physical intimacy and tenderness with their spouse.

Although personal spiritual awareness is not the reason these couples chose celibacy as a lifestyle, interpersonal spirituality, an embodied way to include the spiritual dimension of a relationship in the physical love a couple feel for one another is something that Brown , Pearsall and the Tantric practitioners feel is essential to a sustained, satisfying and healthy relationship.

There are many good reasons for this. Spirituality offers us a view, a vehicle, *and a feeling of love.* Crossing traditions, the mystical branches of all faiths have catalogued a myriad of physically ecstatic experiences of love between the disciple and her guru or the believer and his God. These episodes are rivetting of the heart, mind and soul. And all can be boiled down to a simple beginning. Llewellyn Vaughan-Lee after setting a path for the beginner in meditation recapitulates, "rather than attempting to still one's thoughts by focussing on the mind, one focuses instead on the heart *and the feeling of love* within the heart, and thus leaves the mind behind. (Italics mine)"[xxi] Many of the saints and mystics in our own Western religious tradition would agree.

"Love and do what you will" (St. Augustine). There is an unusual property to an experience of union with God that reads like sexual union yet it is embodied very differently. An understanding of something called 'psychasm' may give us some clues to this experience of total surrender and union. Grace, it is said, works on nature. "Do whatever moves you most to love" wrote Teresa of Avila.

An intriguing corollary to an application of spirituality that furthers our physical intimacy, is that this brand of physical intimacy might make less rare, what mystics have for centuries been the exclusive guardians of. If we are able to cultivate relationships where we can be naked and surrender our spirits deeply into the arms of another, we might more readily prepare our hearts for the overflowing satisfaction of Divine ecstasy, enlightenment and union.

But we need to engage a context that might be foreign to our lived understanding. The Song of Songs is an example of favored reading by Western mystics yet to simply call the text "sexual" includes an array of explicit sexual or erotic behavior that is not necessarily conducive to deeper feelings of love or mysticism. "His left hand is under my head, his right embraces me" (8:3 Song of Songs) is placed in one context when it is like the woman in my introduction who held her friend and was tenderly and powerfully moved by the embrace, and quite another when it is placed in a possessive, erotic context.

There are then two possible contexts. The first one is what we are currently familiar with. It is a sexual context where something I will call "tenderness" is rare or incidental to our significant and loving relationships. It reflects suspicion onto all of our affective bonds and maintains a distance of safe non-touch. These relationships are deficient in (for –itself) tender touch, and if these occur they are within a relationship that demands sexual commitment. Because of this commitment, there is no possibility of unconditional love. And where the act of marriage and the goal of relationship are sexual, there being no other definition that identifies marriage from friendship, fathers and husbands are given a very small script to play.

Women are breaking off more romances and marriages than men. For those professionals in the family therapy fields it is common knowledge that marriage and the raising of children are a formula for depression for women. On the other hand, it is a formula for good health for men.

Conservatives and Church authorities might argue that the cause of the world's ills are artificial contraception and abortion, which invite men to be more sexually irresponsible and coercive of women. But in fact, it is patriarchal structures that have placed sex and its procreative form at the definitive core of marriage. Marriages must be consummated in order to exist at all, and sex is seen as the place of "union" in the relationship.

On all levels of our society, nonprocreative penetrative intercourse is not labeled as the irresponsible act that it is. Boys will be boys, and men are never discouraged to play the field or gain experience before marriage. We promulgate the myth of "safe" sex and when it isn't safe, we offer a laundry list of trauma remedies to choose from. And when it forces a moral woman to undergo an abortion with all of its subsequent trauma in order to save her life, we as Church excommunicate her instead of taking responsibility for her moral and intimate dilemma or even offering her a shoulder to cry on.[xxii]

A tender context for our deeply involving relationships would have sexual congress as incidental component and not a primary one. Interpersonal sex would continue to be regarded as natural, God given and healthy, but would not be given the absolute priority in our relationships that it now has. Tender lovemaking could be widely taught and offered as a serious alternative to a one way or no way code of living. And far from frustrating its participants, it would relax and relieve many of the tensions and stresses of contemporary living in a society of rampant sexual myths and mores. Finally, there will be the space within physical relationships for genuine, self-sustaining intimacy.

Most importantly, there will be freedom for greater intimacy without added repression, and without the sacrifice of broken bonds and tortured choices. We have found a new adhesive for the crumbling structures of paradigms and roles that can no longer hold and define its participants; and it is only as painful as tender love.

Transition to new understanding

Due to a sexual climate of repression, reverse repression and guilt, we turn inward to our dreams and fantasies for validation and release. In spite of a global effort to release sexual behavior from its secrecy and shame, the vast majority of persons continue to feel guilt and low esteem over incidents as common as masturbation. But now, the person consumed by a desire to masturbate or engage in other sex acts, may feel guilty also about feeling ashamed.

The discomfort is only exacerbated by a view of sex, sexuality and intimacy as somehow inclusive of one another. As the Whiteheads reflect, "We can picture their relationship in three concentric circles. In this image, the smallest circle is the realm of sex. Sexuality, the next larger circle, holds within it the experience of sex but includes more. The largest circle, intimacy, takes in the realms of sex and sexuality but goes beyond to include other kinds of closeness."[xxiii]

Although intimacy can certainly be brought into our times of sexual congress, it is wishful to submerge all sex concentrically

16

within intimacy. For all intents and purposes, widening our understanding of sexuality to include our emotions and other forms of physical closeness has not sanctioned the redemption of our sexual behavior from guilt and repression. Instead, what has become an almost interchangeability of terms between sex, sexuality and intimacy has led to confusion and suspicion with a lessening of nongenital physical closeness in our society.

At the root of the problem is something that is commonly referred to as dualism. A patriarchal church and Judeo-Christian tradition have laid down a perspective and code of living which presume that the mind is superior to the body. And the spirit is an elevated, lofty and pure expression devoid of either mind or body, but especially lacking bodily urges or influence. The sexual revolution, feminism, and new ways of understanding physical intimacy have sought to resurrect the body and women, who as a group have been associated as the source of a man's bodily temptations. But instead of uniting the body, mind and spirit in a new way, the literature only clumps the same hierarchy in a new, positive light. Both, unfortunately, are erroneous and deluded.

The ongoing dialogue and commentaries on the Song of Songs are a prime example. The Whiteheads remark, "Nearly all Jewish and Christian interpreters have viewed this poem as an allegory, describing either God's love for the human soul or Christ's love for the Church. Its message they argue, is about spiritual affection, *not* about human, erotic love! …Only recently have scholars questioned this allegorical "apology" for the Song of Songs. In 1953 the biblical scholar Roland Murphy challenged Cardinal Bea's interpretation, suggesting that the text be taken at face value-not as an extravagant allegory but as a poem in praise of erotic love. Following Murphy's lead, Daniel Lys, Phyllis Trible, and other scholars are helping the Christian community recover this biblical perspective on sexual passion. This recovery encourages contemporary believers to trust their own convictions about the goodness of sexual pleasure."[xxiv]

It is clear that the Whitehead's mean, by their many interpretations of the text of the Song of Songs is that explicit sexual intercourse, begetting children, initiating foreplay, are what is "recovered", by the "goodness" of the passages of the Song. But in fact, this becomes just one more allegory, albeit in a new direction.

"His left hand is under my head, his right embraces me" (8:3) When we truly view the text at its face value, it can be like a woman who in our introduction was holding her pregnant friend. In this case, it would be a male who embraces a woman. The scene conjures meaning from the posture of the woman who surrenders to this embrace. It is also moving in the way the woman is held, which for itself, describes him beholding her, comforting and sustaining her. This is an experience that stands beautifully for itself, and reveals dimensions of intimacy all on its own.

Further, we would have to extend the picture in order to reveal the meaning the Whitehead's would prefer. The male would have an erection, and the woman would be inviting in a myriad of ways, perhaps by her hand wrapped about his penis, something explicit. Though this does not alter the goodness or holiness of the passage, it does irrevocably change the brand of intimacy, the level of undifferentiated love, and whether we are viewing passionate love that is unconditional or provocative.

The leap to sexual interpretation while well intentioned, only imprisons the possibilities of such an example of tender expression to stand alone. While it is exactly this type of experience, liberated from an explicit context that frees us from guilt and shame, it continues, within a new dualism, to repress and deny a deeper, and more fulfilling way of love.

We know that the tender, nongenital touch we received as infants is precisely what enables our procreative sexuality to function properly as adults. It is much more reasonable to try a model of human loving which instead of concentric circles, looks more like Mickey Mouse, with tenderness as the body of the face, and sex and sexuality as the ears. In this Venn diagram, the "ears" are given life and energy by the body of the face, but are also enabled to have a life of their own.

According to Freud tenderness was a sublimated sexual urge. Though many trends in psychoanalysis have parted from his thinking, we are still blurring the boundaries of what is something sexual, and what is tender love. The word "sexual" has become an umbrella reference for almost everything that the body is capable of experiencing. The word "tender" is used in and out of a genital context to describe care of an infant on the one hand and then a rich experience of solitary sex in the bathtub on the other.

But there is a world of difference between tender touch in a context of definite or even possible self gratification and a tender encounter that has either no self interest or a surrender of pleasurable expectations at the center of its intentionality. The former in comparison is simply not profound. Sex, true to its root meaning, can be a grim reminder of how cut off and separate we are from others. And any attendant guilt and shame may call out a reversal in direction of loving; instead of allowing our sexual expression to be fueled and nurtured from unconditional tenderness and love, it spins out into its own course, taking a life of its own. Erich Fromm emphasizes, "The awareness of human separation without reunion by love-is the source of shame. It is at the same time the source of guilt and anxiety."[xxv]

The term "making love" is used almost synonymously with sexual intercourse. Such a prevalent and accepted understanding is simply dangerous and reprehensible, and we are suffering for it. The implication is that love and intimacy are only an act away, that we can control and "make" love. It also makes refusal of a sexual encounter, or physical closeness without a genital localization seem crazy or unhealthy. (everyone wants to make love, don't they?) All or nothing, we may only look at another or touch another with love if there is an opening for a sexual coupling to occur. Freud's notions are as much in force today as ever before.

We have moved, not from dualism to a more integrated sexuality, but into another dualistic mindset. In the past the mind was placed in a superior relationship to the body; today, almost the reverse is true. There are universal feelings of confusion regarding our sexuality. It is probably the only experience we can be certain of when we are falling "in love". Instead of letting ourselves become therefore suspicious as to the assumptions and conclusions our society has placed on intimacy, we persist in ever newer pronouncements of expanded sexual behavior and emotional introspection.

The two are never combined. We are instructed by the experts that we are to overcome our discomfort; any feelings of shame or guilt, and to override our own understanding of conscious or unconscious desires and simply do it. We are taught to act out our fantasies with our partner instead of coming to know and love the integrity and reality of their being; to engage in the reading and viewing of explicit materials, and not to express concern or disgust with the pornographic preferences of a spouse. We are encouraged to exploit our emotions and our spirituality in order to enhance a sexual encounter, and to withhold sex only in the interests of nonsexual technique that will "fix" sexual dysfunction.

The dualism becomes entrenched in the body/mind, body/emotions, body/spirit split. In order to cure this cutting off of our mind, emotions and spirit, we must grow in the ability to connect the three. Associations that attempt to liberate, such as linking the feminine/ecological age with an awareness of how we are sensual and sexual beings only brings to a more positive light more ancient connections between femininity and the rape of the earth. The result is a truncated, not integrated view of humanity.

We are not merely sensual/ sexual beings. Our flesh is emotional. We weep and groan and laugh and exult through our bodies. Our bodies are our language. We come to know a person's mind best through the posture and gesture of their body. Finally, our bodies are incarnated spirit. Our flesh and blood is spirit and through the fabric of our bodies we enspirit and make holy the world.

Our intentionality, emotions and spirit all must become a part of any truly loving encounter and any time we are seeking union with another living being. To be fully a part of our created nature is to graze timelessly in awe and wonder of the fullness of its landscape, and not to squeeze ourselves through a portal of fantasy and fleeting reality.

True integration of body, mind and spirit makes palpable and unmistakable the communication of love and spirit to another. So much that we are never left to wonder what was on our partner's mind the morning after.

Tenderness

Some years ago, after coming out of a spiritual direction session, my director offered to embrace the pain I was feeling due to a personal crisis I was weathering at the time. My circumstances were so traumatic, and her offer so humble, that I received her embrace. The rest seemed to be in slow motion. I stayed within her arms for an extended period of time; and longer still, out of trust for the person I had come to know. Years later, I remember vividly the conscious decision, the "oh, what the heck, I really need this and its ok", of placing my head on her shoulder.   Completely then, my weary spirit surrendered and opened into her comfort, into her compassionate form.

Afterwards I reflected on the power of the experience; I was overwhelmed by love, comfort and acceptance. Among these feelings which were stirred in me, I was dimly reminded of when as a very young child I was held in my mother's arms. I became aware of a level of intimacy which was deeper and more powerful than any physical encounter I had ever known, including many varied and happy sexual ones. The *untergang* or surrender of trust I made also became a component in my personal meditation times. In prayer the soothing effect of descending or letting go into a bath of God's compassion provided a powerful and satisfying *Other* to the presence of my friend. Although the Person was different, the path was the same.

From birth, as infants and toddlers we communicate with our environment and with others in very physical and natural ways. Touch and the desire to be held IS our communication with the world. At around the age of five or six however, we begin to learn the complicated proscriptions of holding back and in, and how to feel ashamed of our needs for closeness. Our innocent bodies are taught that our touch has sexual/genital connotations and that we now must deprive ourselves of physical intimacy until such time that we find a sexual partner. Then we must be satisfied with sex and sex alone, and this is only to be experienced (so the marriage myth works) with one person.

When my first child was born I felt so overwhelmed by the affectional possibilities, that I became concerned if I might be touching and kissing my baby too much. My mother's response was gratefully authoritative. You can never touch a child too much! My son, who is more kinesthetic than my daughter, up until the age of twelve was often inclined to climb in front of me, spoon fashion, on the couch if I came into the room to watch television. I was his favorite, comfortable chair. And at nighttime, after reading a story or singing to them both, caressing them and leaning over them to kiss and hug them 'goodnight' I would invariably be caught in a tender tug of war once their longings for closeness were activated; and they would not let me go!

It is not rational to think that the very essential ingredient to our emotional and physical wellbeing as children can suddenly be dispensed with or rigidly controlled without harm or frustration. We never outgrow longings for physical closeness that are as innocent and satisfying (more so even) as when we toddled into and over our parents' laps. As adults this lack of trusted nonsexual, unconditional love and affection begins to take its toll on our emotional and physical well being; and where the harsh realities and stresses of life are met bereft of mother nature's insulating warmth, we begin to scar and bend and ache with longing.

For males, the cultural taboos pertaining to nonsexual touch are stronger than those for women and can be particularly limiting on different levels. The author of *Consious Loving* notes:

"...as I overcame this old program and learned to give and receive touch more freely, I noticed several profound shifts. First, I became more in touch with my feelings. Letting myself be touched caused something to relax inside, which allowed me more access to myself. Second, my physical skin, which had always been dry and rough, became much healthier. The third change, which I know intuitively but cannot document, was that I got more healthy in general. I used to get several colds a year, often with the change of seasons. Now I rarely get even a mild case of sniffles. I can remember only one cold in the past decade...It has been proved to my satisfaction what a lot of studies have shown - touch equals health."[xxvi]

Once we successfully cork our needs for soothing touch, it is no surprise that we reach for a wide range of assuaging substitutes. Therapists, chiropractors, and physicians provide a substitute for unconditional care and bodily concern. The search for God (and love) is a booming industry where we seek to understand and bring closer the same comforting Presence that was for most of us readily communicated as infants. In meditation and spiritual books, manuals, tapes and workshops we try to calm and reclaim our lives from the countless stresses and traumas we have been subjected to over the years. Other outlets, such as alcohol, marijuana and cigarettes fulfill the need for calm without the painful work of self awareness and integration. The one place where we are allowed to express any physical needs, sex, becomes overburdened, and we therefore become confused as to the place where pleasurable intimacy ends and erotic titilation begins.

If intimacy or sexuality dysfunctions, or if we want to deepen these areas of our lives, the list of cures reads like activity we might find in a nursery. Nonsexual touch heads the list. Others include sitting or lying together spoon fashion prior to a sexual encounter in order to "improve sex". In one book entitled *Super Marital Sex,* the author devotes one small chapter out of several hundred pages of explicit sexual material for the recipe of the book's main topic. Out of thirteen suggestions one was neccessarily involving the erotic. The rest involved: listening with care and empathy, nonsexual touch, a bath and massage, reading a book together, and prayer or some form of meditation together.[xxvii]

Outside of whatever comfort we are able to carve from a sexual relationship, as adults we remain tense and at odds with the confining restraints of the outside world. In places where the usual rules of behavior are set aside we feel suspicious, judgmental and inept. A local masseuse writes, "Whenever I have my hands on skin, the primary message I am trying to convey is 'you're safe. Let your edges receive the world, which is kind.' This is an extraordinarily difficult thing to realize. Before the massage begins, I can see it in how people hold their shoulders and heads or their limbs almost off the table, thinking they are relaxed...

I have to teach many people how not to 'help' me give them a massage. If letting the table hold you is difficult, letting another person carry the weight of your head or hand or leg is even more so. I make my clients practice letting go. They are surprised to learn that they are holding on, holding up. It's quite a meditation, learning how to be an infant again, receiving care."[xxviii]

I Wilhem Reich, a pioneer in the development of psychosomatic theory, referred to "character armour" as the bodily traits we manifest over time as a reaction to the fear of unpleasure. As a corrolary to his theory of a perfect orgasm which could only be obtained by the rare individual devoid of any neurosis,

"He found that muscular tensions blocked the spontaneous surrender necessary for the maximum sexual pleasure...Chronic muscular rigidities, together with certain character traits, act like a kind of armour to protect the individual from unpleasure, though at the same time making him less sensitive to pleasure."[xxix]

For Reich, it was the sexual prohibitions and moral codes of his day that posed the problems for the healthy, pleasure seeking adult. So much so, you could see it in the posture, gait and the way they drew a smile.

Our bodies are ALL. Sales and marketing materials draw upon early knowledge about body language. We know that when we are speaking to another person, only 7% of our communication is conveyed through our words. 38% of what is taken in by someone else is through the tone of the speaker's voice. But 55% of what we "say" is via our bodies.[xxx] When we are not orally relating, 100% of what we express is with and within our bodies.

Spiritually as well, God communes with the soul via the body's sensations and we are moved. We are moved by *a feeling of love.* Teresa of Avila writes, "I used unexpectedly to experience a consciousness of the presence of God, of such a kind that I could not possibly doubt that he was within me or that I was wholly engulfed in him...Previously to this, I had experienced a tenderness in devotion, some part of which, I think, can be obtained by one's own efforts. This is a favour neither wholly of sense nor wholly of spirit, but entirely the gift of God."[xxxi] When we have come seeking love or oneness with God in prayer, it is entirely our bodies that feel our longing, and communicate our desire. Teresa of Avila counsels "do whatever moves you most to love". It becomes for us a mandate to know how fully our bodies can be moved and surrendered in love; how that love feels, and how we may allow love and God to completely overcome us.

The path of the saints and mystics, who chronicle their own ecstatic love encounters with the presence of God, show us a way of loving that is much more satisfying than what the physical limitations of an orgasmic climax will allow. In order to understand such a movement, we need to attempt a clearer perception of this kind of embodied surrender into love. What it is, and what it is not.

I will call this way of love "tender" love instead of just plain love. One purpose of this is to set it apart from other articulations of love, such as Scott Peck's, "love is concern for another's spiritual growth."[xxxii] While this description is profoundly applicable to our human relationships, it does not go beyond those boundaries to include our relationship with the divine. That is, we do not in our prayer and meditation come to a loving concern for the spiritual growth of God. Yet love is very much an essential aspect of our relationship with God. Love is God.

Peck's definition also does not address the physical stirrings, which are intrinsic to our communications with neighbor and with God. We evidence here a split between body and soul instead of the necessary communion that exists among the two. The question is, how do we physically demonstrate a care and concern for the *embodied* spiritual growth of another? Put another way, **how do we nurture the growth of *a feeling of love* within others and ourselves?**

We also must embark upon new territory in how we view and define sexual behavior. "Sexuality" has come to represent all embodied experience, from a hot bath to having intercourse. Like a woman who wants to cuddle but is then accused of teasing for more; all that has to do with the body *cannot* be seen as "sexual".

What was once seen as all bad (the body) is now being seen as all good and of highest importance. What was in times gone by a bad tease is now a healthy and necessary one, but the misunderstandings persist. It is still a tease, instead of an experience with its own subtleties and range of affectivity. When we view our sexuality as being one and the same as any and all of our physical longings, then we really have not advanced in any understanding toward our bodies in thousands of years. In spite of our sexual revolution, the real problems and frustrations remain: How do we physically bond in ways that are everlasting and profound? How may we completely irradicate sexual shame in our lives? How can we love tenderly in freedom, without having to be accused of subconscious genital urges?

The sexual revolution has been wonderful in bringing some healthy perspectives to bear on our sexual longings. But because it has assumed that everything we physically experience is sexually rooted or shared, it has not been helpful as we attempt to sort out our feelings; to discern which longings to follow through on, and which to lay aside. Our aim is to deepen, and not to alter (or make sexual) the direction of intimacy, although that is certainly an option once a dialogue and understanding are made clear.

For the purposes of lucid dialogue and as an aid to terminology and straightforward communication, I will only refer to genital expressions and longings as sexual. I will also refer to relationships as sexual if genital behavior is considered a necessary factor in the relationship (i.e. almost all current coupling/married arrangements) and any that are seeking or moving toward that end, such as romantic and possessive or exclusive relationships. The term "erotic" I will use only to denote limited ways of viewing the body in ways that are explicitly sexual, or genitally tinged and motivated. All other forms of embodied expression I will try to describe accordingly, and I will attempt to employ the term "tender" in a consistent fashion for similar, unconditional forms of physical intimacy.

Finally, I will develop some potential guidelines for tenderness. How we can check our relationships, and our own intentions and touch in loving another human being. We have many self help books available to us if we would like to enhance the way we love psychologically and emotionally. We also have access to many spiritual guides and reading materials that can help us to pray and worship in ways that deepen our prayer and meditation. But there are no checks and balances applied to our physical loving in any concrete and integrated way, except to enhance pleasure. Though a correlation between the sexual and the spiritual is often hinted at, there is no real articulation available outside of the standard sex manuals. What is sacred, loving touch? How can we comfort a friend, and hold a child? How can we learn to demonstrate warmth? How can we know that our touch or embrace will continue to comfort long after the experience is over? How can we help prevent our touch from being misunderstood?

There are some exercises that attempt to start persons on the road to experiences that are variously referred to as tantric sex, out of body or mystical sex. Some of these are helpful to this discussion and will be mentioned a bit later on. Although these are actually suggesting a nonorgasmic interchange of physical intimacy, they are offered as a form of sex; and do not offer to differentiate more indepth touch which incorporates tenderness and warmth from the regular ways a couple might touch and behold each other during sexual intercourse. The results, however, are similar to tender lovemaking and are offered as a "risk free" alternative to sex. But the reader needs to be aware that in order to maintain some consistency I will be regarding these forms of "sex" as tenderness, which they really are when found in their purest forms.

Ultimately, we can take these guidelines and make love in a new way; or we can simply use them to enhance and lend confidence to our own embodied communications in a relationship of some physical and emotional distance. Or, we can stretch our souls to their embodied limits; become one with Eternal Being, and enjoy the satisfaction of all desire...

Tenderness: a surrender into Presence.

One man said to me, "I don't have to be passive, do I?" Plainly, no. Tenderness is not about sitting back and simply allowing something to be done. Instead, it is aggressively humble. Tender touch is not like a massage, where one person is receptive, only, and the other is engaged in activity for some purpose, whether it be for the relaxation or enjoyment or pleasure of the other person. Tender movement originates from pure love, from all parts of the body, which are involved in the enactment of this expression. It is a gift of self, without craving or seeking anything in return, and is deeply moving to the recipient when it is correctly recognized as such. Often there is a tender return, and so it goes...

Tenderness is also not about being "touchy feely" or affectionate. There is no Carte Blanche here for indiscriminate touch. Some forms of affection can be simply intrusive to another person. They can demonstrate everything from ownership or authority to personal neediness; and be more of a reflection of someone simply having a good day. This is not to say that some forms of affection are not important or very beneficial. But in tenderness we are reaching out in love that is specifically meant to communicate warmth to the Presence within a particular individual.

Some examples of variety of expression can be found simply in how we say "I love you". There are many ways we notice how shallow and self serving an expression of love can be. Though speaking love is intended to be an offering of something precious and humble, it often comes disguised with many wants and needs instead. The friend who smiles her love with a pleased look on her face and simultaneously reaches for the other person may be expressing her own self aggrandizement, offering a togetherness that is artificial. The individual who simply states his love without strings because something in a recent experience has brought to mind the specialness of his friend, might in fact move his friend and their friendship to a deeper, more tender place.

Thomas Moore writes, "Soul usually thwarts the ego at every step".[xxxiii] A particularly stirring and tender moment is always comprised of a shedding of the ego and a resonance deep within the soul of the other person. Another thought stirring adage, which I am told can be attributed to Jung, is that the opposite of love is power.

Tenderness is also never sexual. One man described an experience where he was alone with a young woman he was seeing at the time. She wanted to have sex with him, but it was her first time, and she was especially nervous. He proceeded at her request very slowly, and became tenderly caught up in the experience. So much so that he was surprised at what happened. He forgot completely about having sex. He felt completely absorbed in their kissing and holding, and could have gone on all night long.

Initially, this concept brings wails and complaints, from those who insist that sex can be tender. Tenderness as a term has from time to time been applied to genital intercourse, but the actual quality of the congress is a layering, not an embodiment of the emotion. Sex can be beautiful, fulfilling, poetic, natural and an array of delights for all dimensions of the body, mind and spirit. It does not have to be tender, as the term and the fullness of the experience are applied here. The other option, is that perhaps a new word needs to be found for what is being described in these pages. But I suspect even then, there would be those who will need to somehow make sex include that as well.

One example would be love scenes from the movie "Shakespeare in Love". While naked, and engaging perhaps in penetration, Shakespeare and his lover recite love poetry from the acts in Romeo and Juliet. This is a beautiful and moving scene, which would capture a tender moment within the whole of the sexual encounter. But once the two began to move toward orgasm, either their words, or the *feeling of love* which was conveyed within their bodies would have to be displaced by the growing arousal. If not, the arousal would not lead to orgasm. It is very much an either or type of phenomenon.

A friend said to me, "But there is something about becoming naked", in order to argue for some special tender qualities that sex has, over and above other forms of expression. But when we view the movie "The Last of the Mohicans" we are reminded that sex is not necessarily about becoming naked! The converse is also true. Our culture implies that becoming naked is irrevocably caught up with the sexual act. In fact becoming naked is all about becoming naked. There is a difference when someone poses naked for an artists' class, for example, and when someone models for the centerfold of Playboy. We may or may not choose to add other, erotic elements to an experience of nakedness. We also may or may not elect to associate other, non erotic, elements into our sexual activity. The reader may notice similarities here in the treatment of the Song of Songs, and the ongoing debate that leaps from one allegory to its opposite instead of leaving it, and finding meaning in its tender scenes, just as they are.

It is sad to realize how much of the many forms of physical intimacy we feel forced to bundle into, and interpret out of, our moments of sexual intercourse. Many women can relate to moments of simply wanting to be close to a man, and being accused of wrongful "teasing" instead. If we removed the pressures of having to fulfill a primary sex instinct; indeed if we didn't think about it at all and simply approached each other with an innocent longing for love and closeness, there would be an enormous arrray of intimate experience opened to our discovery.

Again, I am not at all implying that there is no place for sex in a spiritual and loving existence. Or even, that sex for pleasure only is wrong. But I will suggest that much or most of what we are led to believe are sexual longings are in reality longings for tender closeness. Our sexuality is merely triggered in the process; and because our culture has only genital expressions on our menu for human intimacy we select and nurture these fantasies and desires in the absence of any other alternatives.

Tenderness and nonsexual forms of physical interaction are certainly possible before or after sexual activity, and as we have already found enhances sexual pleasure substantially. The way we touch in order to enjoy a person's body however, is different from the way we offer tender warmth, consolation and reverence. Sexual touch is sometimes referred to as possessive touch, because it is wanting to "own" and manipulate, however subtley, the other's body and responses. We exact from our partner a specific, pleasurable participation that is different from tenderness or affection as usual.

"...we can learn to cue each other in advance when we want to have a night of lovemaking. An arching of the eyebrows, a pat on the backside in the kitchen, a particularly ardent kiss when the other returns, are all cues that we want the closeness and physical release of lovemaking."[xxxiv]

Helen Colton makes these suggestions for differentiation, from what she terms "Body-Centered [or sexual] Touch" and affection, or "Person-Centered Touch [which] is tactile contact that gives to the recipient support, encouragement, congratulations, admiration, affection, thanks, appreciation."[xxxv] Yet a third category we might create for tender touch would be "Presence-Centered Touch". This would be a physical demonstration of warmth, comfort, deep love, reverence and surrender.

In this way of being with another, each touch attempts to be centered in the consciousness of the other. Different from Sartre's description of sexual participation which caresses the other "into their skin", tender touch is slow and nonmethodical. It focusses upon the spirit of the other; the presence of God in the other. Tender touch seeks to resonate and be with the consiousness of the other *where it is to be found*. Each touch proposes to warm, comfort and reverence; finally to surrender into the presence of the other person.

Movement "into the skin" is actually to move away from the goal of tender union. In Eastern spirituality there are some forms of discipline that attempt to achieve a tender type of union, in something called tantric sex:

"Practitioners...remain indefinitely at the plateau (preorgasmic) stage by aligning the rhythm of their breathing with their lover's. When it works, says Sachs, 'you get into this wavelike state that's even bigger than the one produced by having an orgasm. Two people become one. You suddenly feel part of something bigger - like the universe."[xxxvi]

In this procedure, there is sexual touch at the outset and then an attempt to shift from a peripheral concentration to a focus on the other person in a deeper way, by means of their breathing.

But what I am articulating is a way of touching, communicating and being that never needs to begin with sexual touch. With tantric sex, there is a radical shift of the moment of surrender, and a measure of control and manipulation; from first letting go into enormous pleasure, to sudden resonance and giving over to the deeper presence of the other person.

But as in the experience of surrendering into the arms of my friend, the same results can be found in ways that are more direct, and do not require a sexual start.

With some effort, any natural act can be made into a spiritual, loving experience. If we mix a little bit of relaxation and awareness into a good meal, it is enhanced and better digested. According to Marc David, "Awareness cures. Giving attention to eating is the most fundamental level of healing we can reach in our relationship to food. It is also the most rewarding. Experiencing the body brings unimaginable joy and satisfaction, sometimes quiet and subdued, at other times ecstatic and uninhibited."[xxxvii]

A mystical approach to life is able to bring awareness and a personal significance to the most mundane actions of existence by placing their context within a spiritual creation. Julian of Norwich sees the whole picture when she recounts, "A man walks upright, and the food in his body is shut in as if in a well-made purse. When the time of his necessity comes, the purse is opened and then shut again, in most seemly fashion. And it is God who does this, as it is shown when he says that he comes down to us in our humblest needs…For as the body is clad in the cloth, and the flesh in the skin, and the bones in the flesh, and the heart in the trunk, so are we, soul and body, clad and enclosed in the goodness of God."[xxxviii]

Runners also may enjoy a "high" while jogging. And of course, with the application of spiritual awareness sex can be a container for enormous feelings of overflowing spirit, love and satisfaction. But instead of enhancing a limited, physical process, we can actually *become* the spirit and emotion of love in an embodied way. It is the way we can then open ourselves to "Limitless Intimacy": "[Sex as we now know it] can be great, but we often feel a vague dissatisfaction or sense something missing. We long to form a more intimate bond with another and to share an intense, lingering ecstasy...

[Limitless Intimacy] is a total, complete merging of souls that has been described as the ultimate orgasm. The ecstasy we share goes far beyond what we are capable of sharing on a purely physical level...The osmosis of energy we share during spiritual bonding creates unity, a oneness which allows us to recognize that *we are love*." [xxxix] (Emphasis mine)

The Greek word for tenderness is σπλαγχυα (splagchna) or "of the bowels". In the Canticle of Zechariah it is the place from whom Jesus and salvation bursts forth and spills over all humankind

"Through the tender compassion of our God the Dawn from on high shall break upon us. To shine on those who dwell in darkness and the shadow of death, and to guide our feet into the way of peace." (Luke 1:78)

From this tender source comes a man of "splagchnizomai" (Mark 1:40) for whom compassion is within the very fibre of his inner abdomen. In spite of severe moral taboos against touch in the days of the early New Testament, there is no dualism in the man Jesus; who touches women with healing warmth and opens himself publicly to their tender kisses and caresses.

The abdomen can be seen as the seat of tenderness, and is often where tender emotion is felt and nurtured. Like a woman with child, the tender encounter can be carried about for days, with the felt presence of a friend's spirit deep within the bowels. In both Eastern and Western Christian literature the symbol of bearing Christ to others like Mary; or of the womb as a hermitage or Poustinia in Russian, is the way the special presence of God can be carried to the world:

"Applying this example to the mystery of being pregnant with God (and it applies to both men and women), you have, as it were, a *poustinia within you*. It is as if within you there was a little log cabin in which you and Christ were very close; in this attitude you go about your business...It means that within yourselves you have made a room, a log cabin, a secluded place...Because you are more aware of God, because you have been called to listen to him in your inner silence, you can bring him to the street, the party, the meeting, in a very special and powerful way. The power is his, but you have contributed your *fiat*."[xl]

The belly as a place of spiritual power and vitality is called the Hara in Japanese tradition, and is specifically a location in the lower abdomen. The trained practitioner of Shiatsu massage technique is taught therefore to work from the hara, in order to maintain energy and not tire during the body work; and also because pressure from the hara brings control, consideration and sensitivity to their partner.[xli]

In tenderness, there is no need of control, no question of how far to go. We need only to articulate, understand and practice the elements of tender love. These elements are very simple, and extremely natural. There are four important ingredients to tender intimacy: Freedom, Awareness, Reverence and Surrender.

How do you capture another with open hands? Tenderness.

-a new koan.

Freedom. *As we begin, we could practice some letting go. Any nervousness or restlessness can be brought down to rest in the energy of the abdomen by letting gravity gently pull it down. A careful meditation, then, perhaps breathing and watching the feelings that move with the breath is a good process. All agendas, any control, power strata, can be allowed to melt into the breath, and be cleansed into the belly. Now that we have focussed our energy from our hara, and there is only unconditional love moving our touch, we can approach our loved one, tentatively, giving him the space to say "no thanks", or "not there", or " not just that way"...*

If we are not with a partner, in our imagination we can approach our beloved with freedom. Gradually, over time, we can become more and more aware of what we are exacting from our fantasies and let go of them, moving instead into the full reality of our friend's affection. Let the other be purely themselves in our thoughts, without heaping any of our own preferences and desires upon their embodied response. Respectful permission is crucial before touch.

The practice of offering an open hand for shaking began as a way to demonstrate that there were no weapons in the hands and therefore nothing that might be threatening. Open hands is symbolic of having let something go, or put it aside. It is a freeing of the awareness for other less- self- absorbing matters. Blessings are conferred with open hands. Babies are held with open hands, because they are delicate and wriggly.

A spiritual being can never be caught, or coaxed into closeness. The nature of spirit and genuine love is too wild and free for the confines of a romantic or possessive relationship. Only on the surface can an individual appear to be domesticated. Their hearts and souls will always roam free.

It has become a puzzle to marriage counselors, therapists and couples that deep relationships are not always with the one we initially choose out of having fallen in love. Once we are married for a few years, we understand the fallacy of finding the special someone that was meant for us. Indeed, we realize that we could have successfully married any of a score of individuals. Many writers of books on love and relationship blame the falling in love experience, and point to the maturity of realizing that such love is not real. It then becomes part of a stage of intimacy. Real love is said to occur after the high energy of falling in love has dissipated, and the two see and accept the faults and shortcomings of each other.

But in fact, falling in love is part and parcel of the beatific vision of mystical experience, that which is at the heart of deep and powerful loving. It is not really the experience of love that is lacking in our romantic bliss, but our perception of the experience, and how we pursue and nurture that experience. Falling in love is the kiss of God. We continue to fall, and fall and fall through life (if we are open and willing) until we see the One who has been kissing us all along. And then we cry out with

St. Augustine, "late have I loved you!"

When we fall in love with a person, they are in a way, deified. By participation, our own hearts are made larger. We are drawn out of ourselves; our spirits are made noble; and we are ready to love. The problem is that we are not truly free, and we do not necessarily want the other to be free. Psychologically speaking, there are many names for this lack of freedom within an intimate relationship: Past hurts, insecurities with belief systems or habits different from one's own, "baggage", needing certain acts or forms of behavior from the person to validate our own, putting our own judgements on the other's actions, inhibiting and not allowing the other's freedom to express deep emotion or elevating them in ways that we require for our own self worth and ego enhancement.

Consequently, it is our own lack of freedom that chokes love. We fall out of love because we could not endure it, not because we are wise. When we fall in love, we rapidly heap upon the other person a list of criteria, in order to compensate for the enormous call of humility, nobility, vulnerability and risk. One aspect of the other person that is extremely ego gratifying to us is the entertained thought that the other person desires us sexually. That hunch is given strong affirmation and support in our culture. Very quickly then, as long as we fuel our imaginations predominantly with thoughts of the other's sexual response and behavior, the relationship becomes localized and is pursued in that fashion. Initially, the erotic behavior of the couple is fueled internally from the energy of the falling in love experience. But because this energy is not replenished or nurtured, the sex life of the couple, as in our diagram, spins off on its own. Eventually it fizzles. This is our culture's current paradigm for all intimate relationships.

In order to liberate our physical bodies so that we can give ourselves completely in a tender relationship, we must free our perceptions of love from the urgent self-inflicted requirement to act genitally.

Our sexual response is always ready. Women experience lubrication in their vagina throughout the day and several times while they are sleeping. Males also have an erection at regular intervals throughout the night. Studies indicate that these responses have nothing to do with what the person is dreaming about. They simply happen; and because we are calmly unconcerned about what is going on in our genital areas, we do not feel the need to make some sort of urgent or erotic response.

It is very natural to assume that like other organs in our body, the genitalia are capable of an emotional and spiritual response, and not merely an organic, reproductive one. An ability to enhance recognition of these personal responses is essential. The more we are able to slow down our awareness, the more we will be able to pick and choose what our involvement will include.

Some form of meditation both separately, and together as a couple will facilitate the necessary freedom for awareness of scripted programs that have been ingrained in us. Mutual meditation, perhaps while naked, on the breath of the other partner will work well, and later can be a natural way to add power to the love making experience. There are many different types of meditation, yoga and other relaxation techniques and a large industry of literature is dedicated to describing and offering them. Any and all will be effective, not just for intimacy between a couple, but for personal health and well being on all levels.

Unfortunately and fortunately, sexual response is very easily conditioned; and whatever we hold to be true about sex is the way we will continue to act and perform sexually. "it is helpful to get away from the idea that there is a beginning, a middle and an end through which sex progresses. All sexual experiences can be seen as reconditioning or relearning opportunities, and in fact, every sexual experience does influence one's future sex pattern, whether one wants it to or not."[xlii] It is very easy to see how some myths are propagated, especially in the absence or scarcity of adult encounters of physical, nonsexual loves. The predominant myth we must liberate ourselves from as we become close to a person is the notion that sexual urges are the most natural and overshadow any other desires we have toward them.

"In other words, that coming to an orgasmic end is somehow

39

easier or more natural than making love indefinitely, and, consequently, that coitus reservatus involves a kind of fight against this natural force, a holding off, an inhibition, a struggle of sorts, in order for lovers to continue making love."[xliii] ...these myths show themselves to make little sense.

There is agreement among most sex researchers and therapists that sex is a learned, and cultural response. In order to open ourselves to a more powerful and more deeply intimate encounter with someone we must relearn what we have been taught about physical intimacy.

It may be helpful to recall our Venn diagram. It is our capacity for tender intimacy that fuels our ability to fall in love, and our ability to engage in sexual relations. The reverse is not true. We will notice in a later section that couples who are celibate report that they continue to experience the same feelings toward their partner as when they first fell in love. Yet marriage manuals declare that falling out of love with our partner is a natural and necessary part of marriage.

It is similar to being outdoors on a very hot day. When our natural physical selves are being acted upon in such a way that it generates discomfort, we seek to compensate in some way, in the case of sexuality, we take a drink. We have a choice. Staying in the sun, we keep drinking, Since this corrects the problem of thirst. Or, we can go indoors, for a swim, cool our whole body, so that we are satisfied in a different way. Because we all know the difference, many persons choose to go to a cooler place. In matters of sexuality, most of us do not know the feeling of this other option, or that it is a real potential for satisfaction at all.

A friend once remarked that he would not consider having a sexual relationship with his daughter, apart from all of the taboos and the harm it would do to her psychologically. He noticed that a sexual relationship with his daughter would not further, and not increase the depth of feelings he had for her. Similarly, I have had relationships in which the thought of having sexual encounters with someone seemed superfluous and less than what we already enjoyed together. At this level it is easy to see how sex is a limiting and not expansive part of a relationship.

In order to nurture freedom for deeper intimacy in our spaces for physical closeness, we must remember that since about the age of five, we have been unable to fully express our affectional longings and needs. These longings are much deeper and more diffused than any localized sexual desires. Therefore, when we draw close to a person that we love, external social images tantalize and categorize our feelings, so that they become sexually pressurized. Because we can't remember that these were very natural feelings and a part of many feelings of physical closeness when we were quite young, we think we have to push for something sexual.

Gerald May in his book *Will and Spirit* places most of our movements in love and intimacy within an encounter of being *willing*, or being *willful*. Which dynamic and posture we choose when we meet intimacy is reduced to what is simply open to loving, or closed, intent on staying inside of staid, role and culturally enforced boundaries of expected behavior.

Tender touch can only exist in total freedom. It is the opposite of trying to pleasure someone or yourself. It is the opposite of trying to relax someone with a massage. It is not about doing anything at all. It is about freely offering tender love, and allowing the other person to respond freely. Instead of coming up to a friend and throwing your arms around them and giving them a hug for example (making them a rather captive "huggee"), a tender embrace would consist of an open armed invitation; free to receive an answering hug, or not to be slighted (and not to judge) by a refusal to engage in an offered embrace.

The Rosen Method, a form of body work, applies one type of nonpossessive touch that is referred to as "non intrusive". The process is similar to a massage in that one person is more passive, and is being acted upon. The touch is much more gentle, however, and involves considerable interaction with and a coming to know the body and breathing of the client. The Rosen practitioner touches very slowly to feel the various places of the body and may ask without requiring a response, what happened here? This form of shallow touch, has the powerful result of effecting a deeper relaxation, and consequent transformation in the client.

"I started then to understand why relaxation is so powerful, that it's actually the gateway to awareness, the gateway to the unconscious, when we don't hold back. Our experiences sometimes especially when we are younger cannot be handled at that point. In order to put them away, we have this tension in the body. But then, very often we forget about it."[xliv]

Relaxing touch opens our awareness and allows us to be spontaneous and connected to our bodies' real capacity to love in totum. It can be as simple as merely touching tongues or fingertips.

"...and not do anything except feel the sensations. Without "doing" anything or inhibiting themselves, they allow each other's fingers and hands to do exactly what they want to, feeling just what they actually do feel."[xlv]

An important distinction between tender touch and sexual touch is that sexual touch always solicits a response. We are eager for one. Though there is some freedom, our genital sexuality is given within parameters; there is an expectation of specific behaviors and cooperation. Tender touch however, is purely communicative of warmth, love or comfort, has no goal, and is freely offered. Open, gentle and willing, our skin "listens" to the heart of another. Studies of infant care have shown this to foster the most calm and well-adjusted children. For all we know this is the way God in nature births the tiny soul into existence. The gift of love that we can give to someone via our bodies is supreme.

It has been said that there is no greater love than to lay down one's life for a friend. Sometimes the interpretation of this phenomenon is placed within a grandiose scene of literally dying for another person. But in the arms of our loved one, physically, emotionally and spiritually we are put in the rare and wonderful position of offering this deepest and greatest love.

As lofty as all of this appears, an enormous power is right within our bodies. Meditation and other forms of relaxation techniques and yoga are only getting us in touch with what is closer than we are to ourselves. Sometimes, when my own mental and emotional obstacles are too great, I need only to remind myself, in a bit of reverse psychology, that a fountain of love is already inside of myself, and that I am being kept, needlessly from it. Or, I try not to meditate and relax; I think about love, or someone that I love, and try to stay away from feelings of love. Inevitably, in the face of feelings of genuine, tender, unconditional love, other laments are forgotten. Problems seem small and a willingness to receive love and overwhelming feelings of love looms large and immanent.

> *If you understand, things are just as they are. But if you understand, things are just as they are.*

> *a koan*

Awareness. *Once we are able to behold the person toward whom we feel love in freedom, without any of our own agendas, we can bring ourselves within physically intimate proximity. But then, we may feel the tug of nervousness, restless urgings to do something, to begin a rhythm of erotic behavior. All we need to do is stop, and be still, or move so slowly that we are thrown out of any rhythm. Soon, though it may feel like an eternity, our awareness opens. It is like being mesmerized while sitting in front of an open fire or while viewing a mountain range. The body of the other is captivating in new and provocative ways. If we are approaching tender intimacy in our imagination, incredibly, the same experience opens to us. We wait, and it is wonderful.*

Awareness moves us to know in an intimate way. It is about not simply seeing or noticing, with some of our own agenda or colored perceptions but about perceiving an object, person or concept in a very clear way, just as they are. To open our awareness is to be fully conscious. We behold things just as they are.

Unlike sexual or erotic love, tender love does not require the participation of the other and provides freedom for the other to respond. Tender love does not condition its feelings upon the actions of the loved one, and therefore acts without the ego gratification which movement into the skin supplies.

"To summarize, erotic love is characterized by the

43

experience of losing or restricting awareness and has the effect of bolstering self-importance. Agapic love is characterized by losing self-image in bright, open awareness and has the effect -if allowed- of increasing humility. In eroticism, the world seems to fall away. In agape, the world is awesomely present. Yet both are passionate. Both involve immense energy. And both, without doubt, are love."[xlvi]

A view that is nonrestrictive beholds the form of a person in totum. The knee cap is as wonderful as the eyes, the mouth, the breast. All parts of the beloved are humbling in their participation. No area or facet of humanness is ignored or overlooked in its interaction with the whole and the health of the person. Similarly, there is no focus or super importance on select parts of the body over and above others.

In sexual thoughts and encounters the converse is true. We are given to exploring the pleasurable possibilities of narrow locations within the whole range of another person. These erotic areas are exaggerated to a greater or lesser degree depending on our lifestyle, its stresses and priorities. Flipping through an issue of Playboy magazine gives us a clue to how eroticism and sex is a localized encounter. Many of the models actually wear clothing. They are not naked, or natural. Instead, the clothing is cut away to reveal and enhance certain areas of the woman's body. Also, the posing and posturing is very narrow and suggestive of explicit sexual activities or invitations to sex.

Interestingly, it is a preference for a less localized and more diffuse experience, which many men and women will describe when choosing one form of sexual experience over another. For example, while women and men both have stronger and better orgasms in masturbation (either solitary or mutual) or other more genitally focussed sex acts, the majority of individuals prefer the traditional "missionary" position for sex.[xlvii]

Celibate couples make the same comparison when comparing their form of physical lovemaking to a genitally arousing encounter.

"The only real way to be celibate, I believe, is if it's a natural thing. I think your hormonal habits change. If you don't have the localized need, it's easy. In this way, celibacy is more a reflection of an entire way of perceiving the world, a level of consciousness. I can't entirely ignore the sexual messages around me, but I find I can comfortably shift my attention from a lower tug to something more full."[xlviii]

"Now, being together is like making love all the time. That may sound absurd to other couples, but celibacy seems to keep our hearts open to each other. Sort of the way it feels when you first fall in love..."[xlix]

In order to nurture a state of tender awareness when there are feelings of sexuality it is often helpful to simply slow down, slow even to the point of stillness. That may seem awkward at first, because we have not been allowed to be still in someone's arms since we were infants. But after a while, the awkwardness passes and a most amazing thing happens. Our awareness begins to open, and we perceive more than we did before. And all of it feels much more natural, and our movements much more comfortable than we have ever felt before.

At its most basic, tenderness can be seen as protracted touch. When we are touching without movement, for a period of time that is longer than what may be comfortable under normal social circumstances, our awareness naturally opens of its own if we let it. When we are slow, we can move out of old behavior patterns of response and are able to discard any agenda of activity. Our bodies then respond with a powerful energy or ecstasy. The word ecstasy comes from the Greek *ek - stasis* meaning to "stand still". The reason we feel ecstatic is that we are receiving the undiluted voice of God in nature; a message of unconditional love; and overwhelming comfort and joy.

Once our awareness is opened, we can proceed to love more naturally, without the pressures of socially ordained scripts. When we don't feel the pressure to perform in a certain, sexual way, a new view is opened to us, with wholly new and ever unfolding interpretations for our affections. Because this deeper awareness is allowed expression and fulfillment, also freedom from judgements and boundaries, we are able to maintain the state of falling in love. The result is a love that is sweeter, and more tender than sexual love. It is also more rational in its ability to see circumstances in fresh new ways without any of the canned expectations and pressures we have been handed from prior lovemaking scenes (real or imagined).

The amygdala is the portion of the brain that governs all strong emotion, that of fear, anger and also lust. It also is where all of our emotional memories are stored, and is the first place activated for the scanning of a new situation. If we are sufficiently under stress, or are stepping toward a past wound, we may experience a hijacking of sorts by the amygdala. Afterwards, we might wonder at behavior that seemed silly and irrational once we have had the opportunity for calmer reflection.[l]

If our basic lustful desires work themselves into our behavior in a similar way to strong feelings of fear and anger, it is little wonder that we find ourselves in a rut of sexual desire that seems to have a mind of its own. We are not offered any guidance either, in order to rethink our sexual behavior and assumptions. Instead, we are more or less encouraged to "just do it" and not to judge differences in sexual appetites and fantasies. There are many theories of emotional rigidity that can at the same time be applied to our sexuality.

In the theory of Re-evaluation Counseling, Harvey Jackins founds a prescription for health and happiness upon the ability to approach events in a fresh new way. What interferes with this natural tendency to be fully rational are past hurts that have been mis-stored instead of being allowed to heal. These painful scars build within the person and become the many 'buttons' or triggers for chronic irrational approaches to life's challenges.

"Chronic patterns become very 'total' in their effect upon their victims. They are manifested in postures, repetitive cliches of speech, rigid rituals of behavior that are included in the responses to all situations. They include chronic emotional attitudes. These emotional attitudes will become etched upon a person's facial expression in the signs of grief, anxiety, etc., which most older adults wear whenever in 'repose'."[li]

Like Marion Rosen, Jackins believes that healing and transformation of past hurts is possible through the 'discharge' or release of the emotions and feelings surrounding the hurt. Proper healing is facilitated by the attentive presence of another person, who non-intrusively midwifes the uninterrupted flow or discharge of grieving. This person does not merely hear the person's story or trauma. They bring their own body to bear on the experience of the other person in nonsexual ways. The posture of the counselor or practitioner is one of comfort and reassurance. It is reverent of the basic desire and competence of the healing nature within the person.

If the quality of freedom enables the person to embody tender listening, the quality of awareness enables a tender sightedness. It is a new lense which is applied to the body of a friend; even to all of creation. If we practice seeing in this way, and employ the following conditions of reverence and surrender, we lose the tension and frustration of the erotic element in our love relationships:

"When I see attractive women, it's not exactly nothing -I look, but it's an appreciation- almost an aesthetic experience. I once heard a guy say almost that exact same thing about his reaction to beautiful women and at the time, I thought it was bull, but now I know what he meant. The physical desire just doesn't take you over in that overwhelming way, and you can really fully experience the woman's beauty without wanting to 'have' her."[lii]

There are ways to enhance the physically beautiful and loving dimensions of our close relationships without negating or repressing our erotic urges. One way is to utilize our fantasies and daydreams. Our daydreams about someone we love become a script which we ultimately play out, either to the detriment or the blessing of the relationship. If we intentionally dwell upon the other's beauty and our loving response and surrender to that beauty, over time our urgent sexuality is replaced with much larger, and more pleasurably powerful experiences. Orgasm, and the need to arouse ourselves erotically, gives way to a lingering rapture, a deeply fulfilling and soothing variety of response.

Another way is to enhance our non-verbal love communication skills, that is, to fully enter our body in love, and to be fully aware of our beloved:

"One way...is simply to sit across from your partner, perhaps touching casually and gazing into each other's eyes. Become aware of the totality of your sensations, rather than concentrating on one perception...experience your partner's breathing, see your reflection in his eyes, feel the texture of her clothes or skin, smell her hair, become aware of the warmth of his body. Do all these things simultaneously. Experience the whole and all its facets in one eternal moment."[liii]

Over time we are able to fall in love without any attendant erotic impulses. This is how the mystics fall in love with God. But it has only been reserved for the saints and mystics because we are raised with a fear of sexual touch, and that all touch is somehow sexually associated or rooted. We lose sight of the awareness that there are very pleasurable sensations, ecstatic sensations, that can stand alone when we are with someone else. There is a difference between tender and ecstatic sensations and erotic, or urgent ones. If we have ever been choked with emotion, or moved beyond words, when something appears so beautiful that it takes our breath away, then we have experienced the beginnings of ecstasy.

One such mystic, Therese Couderc wrote in her diary, "I saw the word 'goodness' written on every thing." When we fall in love with God or with a person, we see with the vision of an artist or a poet. We see the naked model as a work in progress, and not as an erotic centerfold.

The beatific vision of the mystics begins with the awareness that the cup is half full and not half empty. It is a practice of seeing the positive, of bringing our awareness to bear in ways that see more than our own discomfort and frustration. Accordingly, the beatific vision is seen as transforming and redeeming the original fall from grace in the Garden of Eden. But how? Certainly, the lives of the mystics do not become idyllic once they are in love with God. The answer might be that Eden was not as ideally perfect as our imaginations have led ourselves to believe that it was. Only the vision of positive reality was different.

Before the Fall, 'Yahweh God took the man and settled him in the garden of Eden to cultivate and take care of it' (Genesis 2: 15) John Aurelio candidly notices, "It was not perfect. Adam did not walk around in idyllic leisure. In fact, he had to work…if Adam and Eve were totally happy, then there would be no room for improvement. If there were no problems in Paradise, what did the mosquitoes do?"[liv]

All at once, Adam and Eve saw that they were naked (and something needed to be done about it). What we can do, is to see that we are naked (and that we don't have to "do" anything).

> **Reverence.** *Now that your beloved and you are free, and standing still in the awareness of each other, you begin to sense the thoughts and feelings of your partner. Remember that God or the divine is within both you and your partner. Your touch becomes transformed to a caress of devotion and worship. This is the opportunity to not only let your partner know how enormous is the power within them, but also to validate this power, and to draw close to this power of God. How huge, to really have God standing before us, to be able to kiss the feet, the hands, the breast of God. The feelings are overwhelming, and healing. They stay on your mind for days afterward.*

Reverence is the practice of presence. Unfortunately, reverence has been part of a dichotomy in which we tend to lump everything which is nonphysical. The "sacred" means to be set apart. We have in our patriarchal western religious culture taken this to mean something a part from the sexual, and separated from our bodies' feelings of intimacy.

To the contrary, sex with a sense of the sacredness of genital intercourse enhances the way a couple may encounter each other, and can make the experience more intensely pleasurable.

And when we go even farther and embody real tender reverence in the beholding of God in someone we love, and are reverenced in turn, we experience a power beyond anything. It is how as mystics, our bodies pray in the raw:

"For us, contemplation is the contemplation of a Person. We contemplate God as two lovers contemplate each other on park benches, and when they are alone. They hold hands and look deep into each other's eyes. For us, prayer is like a woman contemplating her husband after the marriage act. Both lie still and gaze upon each other in silence."[lv]

Many of us have an inkling of this power if we have ever enjoyed a spiritual friendship,

"Between Christians who pray there is a magnetic field: an attraction more powerful than any merely human passion, but like human passion. The passion drives us to holiness. That is its distinguishing mark.

Between Christians of opposite sexes the sudden intensity of this friendship-the white heat- may be terrifying at first. It is like an eros, so like the drive that makes us want to throw everything over, every commitment, every fidelity, in behalf of simple concentration on or dwelling on the other person."[lvi]

At first, it can be easy to confuse tender intimacy with many other forms of sexual consciousness and intimacy. There are three windows, so to speak of physical intimacy. The most basic and familiar is that one in which there is goal-oriented sex, but the individuals involved do enjoy a sense of the sacred, within each other and within the sex act. There is a comfort in each other's body, and separately in their own. Sometimes, there is a lingering feeling of love. At other times, during an increase of faith, hope or love, the sexual encounter might become enhanced in its physical sensations and sense of spirit. But the feelings are not embodied, per se, and are more incidental or layered on top of the sexual program of erotic encounter with the goal of orgasm.

It is like a walk in the woods, where we feel a special part of nature and higher joy in being amid nature. We pat and admire the majesty of an oak tree and the stories this old tree could tell. We see nature as the handiwork of God and may or may not enjoy a unitive experience of special harmony; but we do not walk in order to experience God directly, or see God everywhere in nature.

The second way of sexual intimacy is to harness the energies of foreplay and arousal in order to celebrate the spiritual affection and intimacy between a couple. The encounter is without beginning or end, and ejaculation is not encouraged. Each get together is couched within ritual and the spirituality that is seen by the couple for each other. This is similar to Pearsall's concept of "psyche-asm", and is a popular throwback to Tantric practice. Here, communication is at a premium.

All nature is regarded as sacred. We click with the spiritual consciousness in which our partner is imbued. We behold nature and our friend as a holy vessel, and move in this fashion when we interact. Our touch confers blessing, and our kiss reveres the temple of the Holy Spirit. In this mode we cannot grasp, grab, squeeze, pat or caress in a purely erotic fashion. Revealed instead is a deeper power and fulfillment, the "wavelike state" mentioned earlier in a successful act of Tantric sex. We cannot think of two things at once. In order to forestall an orgasm, the Tantric practitioner is encouraged to focus upon the light within themselves or their partner.

The last option, is the practice of the Presence of God. For Roman Catholics, it is like the difference between bread and wine as a symbol of the presence of the Christ, and *eucharistia* as the real presence of Jesus. It is the final frontier; where we begin to taste of love that is without measure.

Here, back to our walk in the woods, we are stopped dead in our tracks. We are filled with awe and wonder and are moved at the level of our being. We are accepted. We are not alone. The dawn from on high breaks upon us, and our feet are led into the way of peace. (Canticle of Zechariah)

In the first option of natural, loving sex, we bring the different consciousness of the other person into their pleasurable behavior and attempt to make our behavior similar to theirs, thereby attaining a union of desire and purpose. (This is something in a world where everyone seems to be off and busy in different directions.) In the second option, we have the first option open, but choose instead to focus, not on peripheral desires, but on the real unique consciousness of the other, so we work out of the window of communication. In the third window, it is our mutual rapt attention, reverance, and comfort, that provides the channel for discovery and union of consciousness.

"We reach this different and wonderful level of orgasm by re-entering the spiritual paradise from which we came - a paradise that we were very close to as small children, and perhaps closest to in our mother's womb. Spiritual bonding is like the intimacy and peace we have all experienced in the womb. But it is so much more because it includes aspects of freedom, separateness and ecstasy beyond compare."[lvii]

In the third window, we see God in the presence of our friend.

One overflowing fountain is brought to another and here is where union occurs. We make love to the presence of God in the other, and we are overcome by the love of God expressed in the other. Because this is one and the same Consciousness, there are no more foreign elements. There are no differences at all. "Like a deer that longs for running streams"(psalm42:1), we long for God. Then, we act within the window of the presence of God, and we see that we *are* water. We know God flowing and loving in us, and we feel the presence of God in us and in our beloved. We draw the water inside us, and pour God into our friend. We simultaneously long to drink and feel filled to overflowing.

There is but one temple in the universe and that is the human body. Nothing is holier than that high form. We touch heaven when we touch the human body.
-Thomas Carlyle

Surrender. *Probably, this is incidental to the qualities we have already described. It is a natural outcome of the other three. There are so many feelings and emotions and persons that we can surrender into. In this case, we are surrendering into the presence of each other and the presence of God. We surrender in order to allow the feelings of love and ecstasy to grow inside of ourselves, and to move ourselves toward complete union. The sweetness and comfort this brings us resolves all tensions and frustrations and feelings of separateness. Calm and love overcome us.*

Surrender is that state where we allow someone or something to overtake us. We allow ourselves to be overcome. When that which invites us to be overcome is overwhelming pleasure, love or joy, we might exclaim "huh!" on an inward breath. This is the preorgiastic moment. It is also the pathway to complete and lasting union with a person or with God.

The theory in both eastern and western religious and psychological literature is that all tender consciousness is rooted in one primary sexual energy. If we desire to engage in something other than sexual intercourse, we must therefore transmute or sublimate our stronger sexual pulses into higher forms of consciousness. This really is not the truth of our early existance. We are early on recipients of wonderful forms of nonsexual love. It is only later on, after about the age of five or six, that we learn to deny our tender longings and that these "sexual pulses" begin to take over and dominate our energies. It is not necessary to transmute anything. We only need to slow down, become aware of our nonsexual physical longings and reclaim what has been a part of our primitive as well as our higher consciousness all along.

Elizabeth Haich describes in her book *Sexual Energy and Yoga*, that since all life comes from sex, all energies are based in one primary sexual energy. This is really a view that is dominated functionally by the male sexual response. As we have already seen, a woman need not be erotically involved in intercourse in order to have sex, and need not be erotically involved in order to conceive. In fact, most women do not orgasm regularly during sexual intercourse. Though it may be accurate to say all life must involve male penetration and ejaculation, it is not reflective of the reality of the experience to say that male ejaculation is the paradigm upon which we may base a theory of primary sexual energy for everyone.

Though it is not as easy and straightforward, we could however notice that all life does proceed from some form of surrender. Whether that surrender be a feminine response of opening to the sexual desires of a male, or whether it be the surrender during the preorgasmic moment for either a man or a woman. Science has been scratching its head over why Nature does not require orgasm for a woman to conceive. It seems so unfair, doesn't it?

But it isn't unfair if we are open to the possibilities that maybe sex and orgasm are not the source and root of all life and life's energies. It is feasible that surrender and not sex is the path of life. It is the gateway to both death and life, sex and love, the human and the Divine.

In Tantric Yoga, there are exercises which utilize this preorgasmic threshold, stretching it out sometimes indefinitely, (or until the Tantrist passes out!) [lviii] The Maithuna ritual prescribes an 8 minute interval for arousal and then 32 minutes of maintaining the preorgasmic peak. The couple then separate for more ritual and may or may not complete their orgasm later.[lix]

The Tantric exercise provides us with a good diagram of how the "huh!" surrender is a free response. Unlike eating, where we merely ingest food and our bodies complete the process with digestion, sex and orgasm do not simply carry out their own physiological course once we are aroused. The Tantrist guru explains:

"The paradox in Maithuna meditation is that the turn-on must be maintained while not thinking about it. Many workers simply concentrate on a single-pointed white light; others draw a very complex mandala or diagram and concentrate on each aspect of it. The guru recommends concentrating on a white light or on the intertwined red and gold spirals near the spine. You start to concentrate on the white light when you are near orgasm, enjoying all the pleasurable sensations, all the things that are happening to you. Only when you come close to orgasm do you use your will to withdraw from it, trying to become one with the partner, and one with the light."[lx]

As we approach orgasm, we are overwhelmed by the pleasurable goodness of our bodies, and we continue to open ourselves and surrender ourselves to it's waves of comforting joy. When we do not stop our process of surrender and give ourselves over to an orgasm we enter back into our bodies to the completion of an electric climax in our organ. Because our physical organs are limited in what sensations they can produce, our experience is also limited within, of course, the range of physical pleasures that are possible.

If we do not enter back into the climax, it is possible to bring the wide open, aware and fully ecstatic "huh!" state into a surrender experience with a person or with God. I am not talking about having sex with God. The arousal is actually superfluous to the "huh!" threshold. Arousal is merely one way of bringing us to a place of feeling overwhelmed by something very, very good. It feels too good to be true...

Similarly, with the other steps we have already mentioned, of Freedom, Awareness and Reverance, we are brought very naturally to this same experience of surrender without the need to push ourselves or anyone else to arousal. Surrender into the unconditionally loving presence of a friend is less limiting because it is not seated in an organ only. Instead the feeling is diffused in an incredible way so that the feeling is like one incessant orgasm, everywhere.

"The great Indian saint Ramakrishna, for example, noted that the penultimate celibate state in yoga 'was one in which it seemed that all the pores of the skin were like female organs and intercourse were taking place over the whole body.'" [lxi]

These descriptions are in sexual language only because our culture has strictly limited its experience of nonsexual love. Like the examples given in the introduction, we are only given a fleeting glimpse of tender love in our lifetimes. In spite of this, the memory and the feelings linger on in our bodies. Imagine if we could give ourselves over tenderly in these relationships, without worry that we have to perform this or that, or change the relationship, or become entangled in expectations. Just imagine if we have had just a tiny experience, what the larger and naked surrender would feel like. Perhaps it would feel too good to be true. That is exactly the path.

The greatest power and knowledge, the greatest flood of overwhelming love, and the most permanent and enduring experience occurs when our surrender is made into the presence of God. Instead of arousing ourselves, St. Teresa of Avila suggests, "do whatever moves you most to love". This exercise also brings us to the "huh!" moment, and to what is often referred to as mystical experience.

The Mystical Chapter

The noblest ministry of nature is to stand as the apparition of God. It is the organ through which the universal spirit speaks to the individual, and strives to lead back the individual to it.
-Emerson, "Nature"

It could be said that there are two powers in the universe. One would be the power of Being or Nature, and the other that power which acts upon Nature. Both are good, both are in God, and both are corruptible. They have various corollaries and dimensions, and the powers play themselves out differently in each of the social and spiritual disciplines. As a response, that which is referred to as left - brained, aggressive, anthropocentric, reason, logic, ego or male centered, is offered a solution or alternative of feminism, ecology, creationism, the sensual/sexual, right-brain development, integration, and mysticism.

The problem is that the struggle continues, even worsens. Central to the conflict is the same power being applied to correct its own deficiencies. That power is usually that which acts upon nature. The apparent reason for this, is that the power of Being or Nature is not recognized or articulated as a power at all.

Consequently, many women are alienated from a feminism that appears militant and oversexed, a replica of a male chauvinism which feminist ideals originally set out to combat. A sexual revolution which sought to liberate our bodies from fear, shame and guilt, is now seeing an onslaught of campaigns that condemn the irresponsibility and repercussions of free and random sex. Poverty has become feminized, sexual harassment is a growing concern on school playgrounds, and artists and nonmaterialists continue to starve.

The mystic, who sets out upon a perfection the hallmark of which is the quieting of restless sexual urges is also left without a clear path. So that the letter of William Johnston to a struggling celibate is not entirely reassuring,

"Such is the human condition. And needless to say, contemplatives suffer this like anyone else. Think of Thomas Merton!...

...[in mystical friendship]When the living flame of love becomes very strong, sexual passion falls into the background, becoming less demanding and losing its compulsive dimension.

And yet the struggle for chaste love is a great one. Consummate mystics have fallen headlong; and some have come to grief. In all this we rely on God's grace which gently leads us to states of consciousness which human reasoning cannot understand or fathom."[lxii]

The contemplative is a seeker of embodied, or mystical experience. With regular meditation in the form of transcendence, the prayer is able to carefully negotiate a route within their own body that beckons full union. This happens by many means; *koinia*, the Greek word for emptying, or Meister Eckart's Via Negativa are some examples. The idea is that if the aggressive passions are quieted, then the presence of God can be felt.

We go to our rooms, surround ourselves with quiet and wait. Or we immerse our intellect into our heart and see God. In any event, the power is one of removing ourselves from Nature and Being, in order to somehow enjoy a fuller view of it. Tension is dealt with there, away from it all. Anger and fear are faced and resolved in the silence where God and transformation are found.

Look but don't touch is the rule. Without feeling our way, we gaze and gaze at love until our bodies are so aflame with raw undifferentiated longing that with risk and a little desperation it is directed to the presence of God. From the inside out, we transcend our bodies until we surrender our bodies back to God, reconnecting ourselves to primal and original energy.

Once back in the marketplace, we are quite capable of transcending every person we meet, until we fall in love. It is then no longer possible to look and not feel. And there is simply not enough time and energy to meditate our way through such a relationship. Our route, which works for our own body, crumbles when applied to someone else's.

And if we are not falling in love, we are the losers. Contrary to popular belief, this is not a safe and mature way to be, even if we are so called happily married or coupled.

While mystical experience ensures absolute ease and certitude with our own bodies and place in the world, we can come to an impasse when our bodies interconnect with a beloved, who cannot be kept at a meditative distance forever.

The experienced prayer can be comfortable in silence and has learned how to listen. With a friend, the contemplative can penetrate the discomfort of any lull in conversation with ease. Two soulmates can enjoy the quiet of a sunset, or just be still, without feeling an awkward need to break the silence or entertain one another with dialogue.

It is harder to imagine close friends who can apply these same skills to their bodies; who can sit, consciously touching one another with feelings of love; apart from any romantic or sexual intentions; outside of any romantic or sexual relationship or even the remote possibility. And beyond the structure of a carefully controlled workshop or contract.

To just be, near and touching one another, without any restless needs to "do something" or "go somewhere" with our touch, is that which invites deepest prayer and union. It is this same route, which opens and directs our diffused longing to the consciousness of God's presence and becomes an overwhelmingly fulfilling and forever completely satisfying love. We literally begin to touch and be touched by God.

The willful exertion of any medium, be it muscular, emotional, or religious, can never successfully bring resolution and harmony with Being. Consequently, even if temporary success is achieved, transcendence, or sublimated celibacy (a sexual power) cannot be brought to bear against eroticism, and religious asceticism cannot insure an uncomplicated and Natural life. Indeed, bringing one and the same power against itself, over and over again, ensures the viscous cycle of one power, outside of the original good harmony with the other power of Being, to run amok.

The only way to return ourselves to the original harmony from which we emerged as infants, is to reacquaint ourselves with the power of Being and Nature. For this to be accomplished, we must not only see God in Nature, or see ourselves as part of Nature, but we must see that We ARE Nature. Once this happens, life is immediately and majestically realigned. In Western Christianity, Mary is able to announce this new order once the Being and Nature of Jesus has begun to take shape within her womb,

> *My soul proclaims the greatness of the Lord and my spirit exults in God my savior; because he has looked upon his lowly handmaid.*
>
> *...He has shown the power of his arm, he has routed the proud of heart.*
>
> *He has pulled down princes from their thrones and exalted the lowly.*
>
> *The hungry he has filled with good things, the rich sent empty away.*
>
> (Luke 1:51-53; *The Jerusalem Bible*)

At the breaking in of pure Nature and Being we are left trembling and overwhelmed by the largesse of God. By "pure" I intend to mean that which has been given in an unaltered or untouched form, but also in a way that is entire of itself and wholly direct, unmediated and complete in its transmission. It is unearned; and we glimpse or gape unconditional love.

Once, some friends and myself attended an evening concert during which we were surprised to discover, a blanket of snow had fallen over the main streets of the town. Spontaneously we decided to walk downtown at what was a very late and deserted hour. The scene that lay before us was singularly enchanting. Not a soul in sight, we were alone amid the virgin snow and streetlights. At one square, lamps with frosted, glassy domes that ringed the park benches beamed swaths of glistening snowflakes which casually danced through the light and the night and our visages. We moved very slowly, turning about with dazed and delighted looks. That night became a chapter on our souls. Without exception, each of us later declared it to be the best time we had enjoyed in a very long while.

At the birth of his son, a friend shared how overwhelmed

with love he felt. Wondering out loud, he offered that while he certainly loves his wife, this brand of love that he feels for his son is altogether different, deeper and stronger...

These stories have very different settings. Yet there are kernels of identity that they share in common. Nature is clearly present, without intervention. Nature is surrendering itself, wholeheartedly, to the beholder. And if the snow could have been personalized, "gift-tagged" just for the individuals standing by, then they too, would have felt overwhelmed by love. The infant son in his fresh completeness declares yet undetracted intimacy and joy. A clean, pink slate; and his tag reads "For Father".

In both experiences, we enter upon a way of being that is devoid of marketing. There is no package, no art. No craft or cunning in order to pleasure or attract. And the recipient cannot lay a hold on a strand of it. There is no way to earn or deserve such a gift. And the converse is the greatest of all. Every fool, sinner and murderer is equally, and well, received of these treasures.

That means us. On any given day, we are given a taste of a goodness that is unsoiled by anything; ourselves. We are forgiven, accepted; consoled. Can we behold the beauty of a flower? Can we feel one with Nature? When we realize that we have been sliced from the same beauty as the flower, that we are inherently whole and complete just as we are, then we can transform any part of ourselves that might seem ugly. A tension in our neck can melt if we place our pain in this awareness. Loneliness and isolation can be transplaced with nurture and belonging if we open ourselves to what F. Scott Fitzgerald named "the fresh green breast of the new world".

Once on a camping trip, my children and I explored the canyon of a riverbed that was at a very low water level. It was a hot summer day, and as we emerged from a trail along the receded river bank we were met by stockpiles of rounded stones and rock that were temporarily abandoned by the force of the white water. As the kids wandered off, I was left alone, standing with my pants hiked in the middle of the swirling water. I was feeling entirely uncomfortable. Circumstances in my life made me weary and in dire need of refreshment. It was also the first day of my menstruation cycle, and I was feeling achy and unkempt in the midst of the heat. The tiny bit of water moving between my ankles felt like a cruel tease. I was drawn however, to the immensity of smoothed stone and rock all around me. It felt incongruous to the water. I stilled myself, and attempted some halfhearted reflections and connections: water as power smoothing the rough surfaces of the minerals; water as symbol of feminine and Mother Nature...

It remained unsatisfying; distracted by the heat and my own discomfort I stood, gazing at the rock, then the water, aware of my own beading perspiration and cramping. Slowly, the unity of Being surrounded and penetrated me. I then became aware without words, how perspiration is water; my period is cleansing my belly; the power of the water is in the rock, and on my brow and within my abdomen. "Washed and clean" resurrected from my spirit. Over and over, with welling emotion, came the resounding "washed and clean".

Thoreau wrote, "What would become of us if we walked only in a garden or a mall?"[lxiii] Indeed, the less manicured a scene, the better; the better to recognize that we have done nothing to warrant the beauty of the land; and without interruptions, the clearer speaks the voice of God in Nature. What has become of us? Thoreau would regard our parks as garden-like compared to the woods or the fields. And a sense of Wilderness, an intimacy with which has vanished with the Frontier, can only make us wonder at what must have been the sheer magnitude of breaking grace.

"What seems to have made the deepest - indeed, indelible - impression, on both explorers and settlers in the beginning, was simply the morning freshness of the continent...the quintessence of virgin nature...that wild freshness. What it offered to us was a chance for renewal."[lxiv]

Perhaps it was the wild freshness that not only drew John Muir into the Sierra, but moved him to embody his environment in mystical fashion:

"Drinking this champagne water is pure pleasure, so is breathing the living air, and every movement of the limbs is pleasure, while the whole body seems to feel beauty when exposed to it as it feels a campfire or sunshine, entering not by the eyes alone, but equally through all one's flesh like radiant heat, making a passionate ecstatic pleasure-glow not explainable."[lxv]

What has become of us? We must find our wildness in the garden and the mall, seeking its source; Julian of Norwich assures us that "All will be well, and you will see it yourself, that every kind of thing will be well."[lxvi] Something green is ever springing up, as Gerard Manley Hopkins brings us back to mind,

> "And for all this, nature is never spent;
> There lives the dearest freshness deep down things;
> And though the last lights off the black West went
> Oh, morning, and the brown brink eastward, springs-
> Because the Holy Ghost over the bent World broods
> with warm breast and with ah! bright wings. "

We come to a juncture. Wilderness is beyond the parameters of contemporary living. Our experience of Nature and Being is limited and rare. Tradition teaches us to somehow transmute or sublimate our sexual energy in order to arrive at overwhelming love and certitude. There are very few mystics. And those who do enjoy mystical experience often find this occurring in their older, retirement years. They often experience the realization that they could have come to this fulfillment much sooner, if only...

It is an affair of the heart. Our sexual energies are given so much practice that we are infants when it comes to an embodiment of tender energies. We are familiar with laughter that is so strong we call it sidesplitting. We know the difference between becoming a little moist with emotion and breaking down in sobs. But we don't have a name or a common experience for a completely overwhelming, life altering experience of pure, tender love that fills and pleasures every pore of our bodies. More than a smile, more than moist, our entire body pulsates with the ecstasy of receiving the love presence/consciousness of an other deeply inside of ourselves.

We reserve knowledge about these things to a few mystics,

many of whom have lived very painful and ascetic lives. To seriously think that this is the way it must be, is to consider God to be very cruel. God is love, yet God reserves overwhelming love and pleasure for rare persons in rare moments in history and only after a lifetime of hard psychological work and interior soul labor? God is like a motherhen, longing to gather her chicks under her wings (Matt 23: 37 *New American Bible*) Wouldn't a mother long to pour soul satisfying love and consolation onto her children immediately and unconditionally? How much more would God! Truly, if there is a God, then our fulfillment and happiness is well within our grasp. We have only forgotten how to open ourselves to receive it.

But the path is still within us ready to be activated, ready to be rejoined to its longing. It is a matter of seeing the world and one another as personal, precious love gift. In this way it is very simple, it is right at hand. Caussade is right when he says "How easy it is to be holy. [holiness consists of] the ready acceptance of all that comes to us at each moment of our lives."[lxvii]

Maybe that sounds like a fairy tale. How can we readily accept the daily horror and violence that go on about us, or even intrude into our lives? Much less, how eagerly do we receive the motorist that cuts us off on the freeway? Caussade is not encouraging a pious form of masochism. It is only when we are in love that the little nuisances of our lives no longer have a hold on us. They just don't seem important. Not that we neglect or ignore our problems, but they are placed in a proper perspective. We can only receive all that comes to us in every instant in direct proportion to how much we love and feel love.

Sometimes a person will say to me, "surrender is too hard for me. It feels too scary, too risky". The best response I can make is "don't do it"! Surrender is not a muscular exercise that we grit our teeth and plunge into. The only time we should ever surrender is when we are totally overwhelmed by love. Then, there are no more vestiges of fear and anger that remain. If there are, then we must sit with these feelings until we can either let them go or let them heal. Remember that we can never push love.

"You surrender when you are in love. It's not merely a

surrender of your body. That's lust. That's a passing thing. That's not a surrender. You surrender to a man or a woman because you love him or her, and then you see that surrender takes on an entirely different meaning. It is equated with love."[lxviii]

Friends have suggested to me that the brand of tenderness I am describing has nothing to do with sex. Hence, Maria, don't trouble yourself with all of this sexual research. Just talk about love. But we have all had the experience of being in a group of persons and sharing something innocently that another individual turns into a sexual joke or innuendo. There is some fun and laughter, and then the conversation turns onto other things. Something is lost, that is the full understanding and expression of the innocent story; and something is gained, that would be a different view of the experience shared, and some lighter moments.

Mystical experience is commonly felt in moments that are accompanied with sexual feelings. Or, we think that what we are feeling must be sexual because it conjures images of physical closeness with another human being. I am not talking about cuddling. I am talking about naked intimacy; but not explicitly erotic feelings. (actually engaging in sex) I am talking about knowing that two persons are in bed together and kissing and not assuming that they are having sex or even trying to have sex. Is that innocent? Exactly!

Mystical union is all about innocence regained. We are talking about something very sweet and tender. Two persons look at one another with love. They keep doing just that. They touch one another without carressing, without movement, only love. Do they feel stupid? Maybe. Because we are encouraged and trained to be about acting on nature, we are always trying to think of something to do. But after some time passes, there is no more awkwardness. They become overwhelmed with love. Their sexual parts may stir. They do not let the conversation become distracted with this. The experience becomes indelible in their hearts.

My son and I watched a video entitled "100 of the greatest touchdowns ever". The criteria for choosing, which of the touchdowns were the greatest, varied, and came down to some arbitrary subjectivity, for which the producers apologized. But the top 10 were decided based upon memory. There are those touchdowns they said, that many years afterward you can still remember where you were, and who you were with when the spectacular play occurred.

It is precisely that degree of momentousness, which accompanies instances of mystical union. When these proliferate, our comings and goings are sprinkled with either direct experiences or memories of great love. We are able to quickly make our own love connections from among our intimate encounters. Life is then one long series of intimate associations.

With all of this huge love to think about at each moment, acceptance of the kind that Caussade speaks of and the surrender that Doherty relates is as natural and easy as eating breakfast. Indeed, having our morning cereal can be a time of being and thanksgiving in the presence of a God who is tenderly and sweetly offering us the goodness of grains and milk to nurture our body very intimately, and personally.

For mystical union to occur, we must give over tender emotions that we once may have thought were reserved for sexual encounters. When we enable this, we can be wildly surprised at what our undistracted love uncovers. Our feelings, to the outsider, may seem sexual. In fact, it is the re - linking of love to our true nature and being. If we did not know the context of his love we might think that John Muir wanted to have a romantic encounter with the Water-Ouzel:

"He is the mountain streams' own darling, the hummingbird of blooming waters, loving rocky ripple-slopes and sheets of foam as a bee loves flowers, as a lark loves sunshine and meadows. Among all the mountain birds, none has cheered me so unfailingly. For both in winter and summer he sings, sweetly, cheerily, independent alike of sunshine and of love, requiring no other inspiration than the stream on which he dwells."[lxix]

Similarly croons Julian:

"And therefore we can with his grace and his help persevere in spiritual contemplation, with endless wonder at this high, surpassing, immeasurable love which our Lord in his goodness has for us; and therefore we may with reverence ask from our lover all that we will, for our natural will is to have God, and God's good will is to have us, and we can never stop willing or loving until we possess him in the fullness of joy."[lxx]

And in the Song of Songs:

"My lover has come down to his garden, to the beds of spice, to browse in the garden and to gather lilies. My lover belongs to me and I to him; he browses among the lilies...

Who is this that comes forth like the dawn, as beautiful as the moon, as resplendent as the sun, as awe-inspiring as bannered troops?" (Song of Songs 6:2,3&10 *New American Bible*)

Freedom, awareness, reverence and surrender. Freedom is not freedom to do as we please, whatever we want, but is a freedom from that which distracts our hearts' desires. That can be confusing when we stand on the threshold of limitless intimacy. Basil Pennington sorts this out within the walls of the monastery.

In this communion of freedom we come to discover the creative energy of love - not as a sentimental or sensual thing, but as a profound, self-giving expression of freedom. [and Thomas Merton] 'What happens is that the separate entity that is you apparently disappears and nothing seems to be left but the pure freedom indistinguishable from infinite freedom, love identified with love. Not two loves, one waiting for the other, striving for the other, seeking for the other, but love loving in freedom'.[lxxi]

When we have true freedom, we are able to unite our love conscious and longing to the love consciousness of another or of God. The original longing we perceived as very young children that was not yet associated with erotic desire is what we are reacquainted with, until we can bring it back to its source; in God or in the love of another person. In freedom, we address the question of how do we foster our mystical awareness? We can transcend nature and our surroundings, or we can immerse ourselves within our being and nature. When this longing is reconnected, or re-linked, we never experience loneliness again. Fear disappears. Anger melts. Did spiders or snakes make you uncomfortable? They will become your friends once this consciousness is rejoined to its source. In paradise regained, to original Being and Nature; we sing our own Magnificat.

Where is sex in all this? It seems incomprehensible that compulsive desire for it might fade. Or that we enjoy something more powerful in its place. But that is exactly how it feels. This is not an exercise in denial or sublimation, which is a "substitute gratification, getting something that is satisfying enough to your desires to relieve at least some of the pressure. "[lxxii] Instead we are giving ourselves over to the fullest experience of the power of love and not a diluted form.

In other words, sex pales in comparison...there is a lot of evidence from the recent research on altered states of consciousness to confirm that: the encounter with the Divinity is overwhelming...It says, ontologically, sexual eros is found in its absolute mode in the Divine Reality - God's passion for the soul."[lxxiii]

The consideration then must follow of sex as a strong sublimation of the more powerful longing and ecstasy of tender union, whether initially transcendant of our physical bodies or immediately belly to belly with a beloved.

The highest spiritual aim does not involve sublimation and genuine acquisition of holiness is far afield of psychic and emotional maneuvers or struggling. In the fourth century this difference was apparent in the stories of the Desert Fathers.

"It was said of an old man that for fifty years he had neither eaten bread nor drunk wine readily. He even said, 'I have destroyed fornication, avarice and vain-glory in myself.' Learning that he had said this, Abba Abraham came and said to him, 'Did you really say that?' He answered, 'Yes.' Then Abba Abraham said to him, 'If you were to find a woman lying on your mat when you entered your cell would you think that it is not a woman?' 'No,' he replied, 'But I should struggle against my thoughts so as not to touch her.' Then Abba Abraham said, 'Then you have not destroyed the passion, but it still lives in you although it is controlled."[lxxiv]

To be sure, when we are in love, sex does not seem to be enough. Our desires drive us deeper, it seems, to a kind of fusion. We long for something more like absorption or osmosis.

Anything less feels like helpless futility, "Like fish at the edges of adjacent tanks, [we] peer hopelessly across into the unattainable element where another has his being"[lxxv]

In this context of enormous longing with a comingling at its source and object, the man Jesus becomes transformed. Tender lovemaking finds its best abode in the God man who lays down his body and spirit to us. "This is my body, given up for you"(Luke22:19), like two logs thrown upon the fire, the flames become indistinguishable one from the other. Consumed with love this divinity with flesh (unaroused) is laid down. Here is the most we can ever be moved with love. It is more than the imagination or fantasy can hold; much more than a newborn son; more than frosted lights on virgin snow. More than cleansed, we are deified and glorified, for no reason at all. Only in a place of tender and mystical understanding can we approach with comprehension the strange words of Jesus, "He who eats my flesh and drinks my blood shall have life eternal"(John 6:54-56).

We are re-linked to the fullest depths of goodness and love right within our own bodies. Consuming and consumed, our mutual elements penetrate; becoming absorbed one into the other. Original nature has been restored and we come home to absolute comfort and joy.

Love Consciousness

Caro Cardo Salutis; The flesh is the hinge of salvation[lxxvi]

If there are two powers in the universe, the power of being or nature and that power which acts upon nature, then there is also a third. The anchor, that is a power that keeps the other two in balance, in wisdom, and in existence was present before creation. It seems to draw us back to original being, and pour us out onto all humankind. The presence of this power is apprehended in none other, than what is commonly occurring in our human flesh, as *a feeling of love*. That power is the power of love consciousness; variously named and personified by mystics of all faiths, and a source of inspiration to great minds and hearts in all mediums and disciplines.

The power of being in nature when we are aware and in

harmony with it, can also be called a Gaia, or earth experience. Daniel Merkur describes this as an 'extraverted mysticism' found in unitive experience in nature. This is as opposed to union within the consciousness of love which is either an 'introverted personal' or 'impersonal' mysticism. A seat of consciousness, which might contain this event, is within an "intense and protracted manifestation of the superego." The superego, the most logical place for such an occurrence "always conveys emotions, ideas, and the impression of a presence that collectively manifests a distinctive intelligence and personality other than the ego within consciousness" [lxxvii]

The superego is a possible source for emotions that result in embodied feelings of love. When recognized and returned toward "the impression of a presence" with an emptying of the ego, union of a mystical nature occurs. We are in love, with another person, or with God. The most important element in this most powerful and tender experience is choice, and mutual choosing. Whenever we are saying 'yes' to God, we may be confident that we have been first, regarded with love, invited and chosen all along.

A mysterious other, imbued with a consciousness which can return or fulfill our longings is intrinsic to the experience. One place we can notice this is in the home, where although we love, we do not *fall in love* with our children. The common phrase, "you cannot choose your family" has some bearing on the love we feel for our family, especially toward those whom we birth into the world.

We are graced with a very intimate physical proximity to our sons and daughters, and as they grow older and develop a consciousness, they begin to separate and become their own independent selves. Looking back upon their parents, there is a discomfort or gap in intimacy, knowing that so much was shared that was not consciously free, mutual and of their own volition.

Nature provides for this 'rebellion of love' in order to spur adulthood and a capacity for fecundity in other spheres of relationship, forming new horizons of family love. In addition to this, of course, there is enormous affection and love that thrives among parents and their children, and this even becomes a model for tender intimacy. It is the love from whom our love source is made known, though we often don't realize it.

We do not have the experience of falling in love with our family, but the presence of *a feeling of love* makes itself known, in ways that can both illumine and surprise. Recently while on vacation in Europe I was overpowered by the miracle of discovering the whereabouts of my half sister whom I had never met. With some trepidation, a cousin contacted her and asked her if she would in fact be interested in meeting me. Her answer was positive, and a correspondence ensued. That Christmas, as I waited for word from my sister, my heart, mind and body were filled with feelings of love. These were overwhelming and were felt no less by my brother. It was a magical and stirring time; of sudden love dawning in our lives.

The reality is that my sister had always been there, it is just that I never knew it. The possibility of intimacy was one that was realized from within my body, a form brought forth from the same father. We knew and shared affection in spite of not knowing the details of each other, perhaps because we did not know more specifics about the other. Nothing formed our awareness except our embodied love.

Love consciousness arises out of the same context. It has been there all along. We are surprised, overwhelmed by love, whether of God, or our beloved. So bodily imbued, we may behold tender love and give over our attention to the gaze of love, and rise to the highest state of consciousness, of mysticism or the *mysterium*. "From each level the subject can break into the mysterium: for example, through the beauty revealed in the sense world on the first level, the subject can break through to the absolute beauty of the mysterium."[lxxviii]

The gaze of this love consciousness as it apprehends beauty needs clarification. The mystical love conciousnes is one which reveals the genuine beauty in another just as it is. It is very different from the false vision that someone might have while in a state of infatuation. It is also not the same as how we see someone who is sexually attractive.

For example, say that we are enamoured of mountains. An infatuated view of a mountain, would be like sitting upon a hill, and declaring what a grand mountain it is, the only, the best, the highest, the most majestic, etc. It is not in touch with reality, although it has the right idea; the proper initial motivation that draws itself out of selfishness and into altruism. But then it becomes derailed. What starts off well, ends up fulfilling personal fantasies and urgencies instead. To outsiders, it is clear, but the infatuated persons cannot see and will not listen. The phrase, "love is blind" is derived not from true love, but from this form of infatuation.

The next way of approaching the beauty of a mountain would be to rank its luster, crevices, streams, height, and surrounding panorama. Ah, the lover would think, the mountain over there is better, I will have more pleasure there. Or, after an initially strong attraction, the lover would notice the faults and failings of the mountain perch, but accept them, resigned to the dullness and corresponding feelings of tepidity but respect and love of the height and depth and other qualities of the mountain. All of these would be similar to a sexual or romantic love.

Love consciousness of a mystical nature is highly aware of the variety within the mountain range and foothills. With gravity and reverence the mountain is held to be not only beautiful but breathtaking, as a part of the Divine presence within creation. The scenery and composite of the heights reveal themselves, without any judgement imposed on them. The shortfalls are seen and recognized, but glorified as natural and becoming to the mountain. Roaming is possible, but it is more important that the particular mountain can receive with appropriate ardor the feelings of love that this consciousness provides. The ensuing gratitude and honor flows out of unconditional love and the result, is the spectacular *noesis* that one is on the tip of an iceberg.

People of course are more than scenery, and when the special gaze of love consciousness falls upon the human likeness, an account reads like the *Song of Songs* (2: 8,9,5,6)"I hear my Beloved, see how he comes leaping on the mountains, bounding over the hills. My beloved is like a gazelle, like a young stag…Feed me with raisin cakes, restore me with apples, for I am sick with love. His left arm is under my head, his right embraces me."(*The Jerusalem Bible*)

Reading the above verses can make one feel frankly warm all over. It is how I experienced them when I meditated upon them while on a religious retreat. At that time my thoughts turned toward how much I was missing my lover, and extended outward from the verses into explicitly sexual imagery. The words of my spiritual director, "you need to be careful when you meditate on this" rang true. But then I wondered if I could bring these feelings of warmth toward a sense of God's presence instead of enhancing the image into one of sexual encounter with my lover?

The successful end result became a milestone in my spiritual journey. What would have been a normal response to these feelings of love was transpierced; the return to me was a reconnection to the source of all love. I say 'reconnected' even though I did not know until then that I had ever been 'unconnected'. Then I was aware of knowledge, whole and of itself.

I remember sitting in the garden later and watching the bees circle close to my feet. I noticed but I did not move; there was no fear. Insight after insight came to me, and I knew that I knew all of it: the purpose of life, of scripture, of earth and humanity. But I could not say exactly what I knew or how I came to know. Sweetness and love were everywhere. A warm presence was in all things. I never felt alone, never bored or restless, never nervous or afraid. Death felt welcome, though I did not seek it, and pain was transformed into joy.

Love consciousness ultimately smashes the mirror of self-consciousness. It cannot be called knowledge in any way with which we are commonly familiar. The Word; perhaps, 'unknowing' is another way to express it. Among Native Americans, who often do not contain a separate word for 'art' in their languages, it might be called a sense of vision with a primal mind. Where "knowledge…that which is so deeply known and felt, so primal in form that it is neither word nor outcry, neither sign nor symbol-but the ineffable thing itself; that which precedes speech and thought, that which is the raw experience itself without evaluation or judgements. It is the ineffable, structured into images."[lxxix]

The special knowledge and consciousness unites and revives a holistic view of the sciences, nature, psychology and religion. As Tor Norretranders posits, an ordinary approach to consciousness comes up lacking, and is the *user illusion*. "Subliminal perception and nonconscious mental activity mean that man's link to the world is far stronger than consciousness suspects...

The beauty of science has often filled scientists with wonder. But the scientific tradition was founded in the attempt to understand the divine principles behind the world. As Julian Jaynes sees it, the origin of science lies in the study of omens, which started in Assyria during the breakdown of the bicameral mind. In ancient Greece, Pythagoras studied mathematics because he wanted to find the divine principle expressed in the world of numbers. The great figures of modern science were deeply motivated religiously: Kepler, Newton, and Einstein. As Jaynes put it, 'Galileo calls mathematics the speech of God'"[lxxx]

Love consciousness is enormous, a pervasive power which when added to the others becomes a triumvirate. Ubiquitous and self-sustaining, these forces are the composite of life. "Drei Kraefte sind im Steine, drei in der Flamme, drei im Worte."[lxxxi] Hildegard of Bingen writes, there are three powers in stones, in a flame, and in a word. They are, for her, different facets of the same God, who is a Trinity.

The glimpse of this love is instantaneous, in physicality, in miraculous gifts, and in personal adoration. So that Rumi can write,

"If anyone asks you how the perfect satisfaction of all our sexual wanting will look, lift your face and say, *Like this*.

When someone mentions the gracefulness of the nightsky, climb up on the roof and dance and say, *Like this*?

If anyone wants to know what 'spirit' is, or what 'God's fragrance' means, lean your head toward him or her. Keep your face there close. *Like this*.

When someone quotes the old poetic image about clouds gradually uncovering the moon, slowly loosen knot by knot the strings of your robe. *Like this*?

If anyone wonders how Jesus raised the dead, don't try to explain the miracle. Kiss me on the lips. *Like this. Like this.*"[lxxxii]

There are also three qualities that identify the power of love consciousness. The first is the tender embodiment of love, as a tincture of the soul within the flesh. Hildegard sees in a vision, "*Denn als Gott die Welt erschaffen wollte, da neigte Er sich herab in der Zärtlichsten Liebe.*"[lxxxiii] (As God desired to create the world, he bent down in the most tender of love.) So that all creation flows and glistens from this origin.

From the German *Schöpfer*, meaning a drawer (of water) is the same word for creator. *Denn die Liebe war im Urgrund dieser Schöpfung schon da, als Gott sprach: Es werde!*[lxxxiv] That is, love was in the original ground of creation already, even as God spoke its becoming. And as God draws forth the soul more and more, the more moist with love, the more perceptible and palpable is the tender love consciousness within a person.

Such a person is like a friend of mine who was in the infirmary of a local religious congregation with Alzheimer's. Over the years, I noticed that information was becoming confused. I stopped hearing from her, and worried that she was in the very state she was. But life was very full, and busy. It was easy to overlook what was a responsibility of love and relationship. And how did that responsibility apply in this relationship, where she might not even know me? Then when I stopped to ask two Sisters from her congregation, they informed me that she was as beautiful as ever. It startled me, to think that she might be the same person, even though her mind was failing her.

Fourteen years prior we met on a religious retreat. It was my first retreat in silence, and when I sat in the dining room with two dozen other women, it felt odd not to talk. I will always remember how my gaze fell on her, and how struck I was by her personal transparency. The beauty of God radiated through her body in such large measure, that she appeared grace filled even in the way she chewed her food.

The following year, I returned to the same retreat and noticed that I was being locked out of the bathroom I was sharing with my suitemate. Finally I went knocking on her door to discover that it was she. A beautiful friendship blossomed from this, even though she continued to forget to unlock my door, the handle of which now sported a yellow lace ribbon. Everyone at the retreat house was aware of her special glow, and it was easy to refer to her in conversation. Instant recognition came with a description of "the brightest, most radiant one present here".

So when these Sisters declared her personal beauty to be unchanged, I garnered some courage, and visited her on Easter Sunday. As I entered her room she turned to greet me, and was clearly greeting someone else, but it did not matter. I felt just as awestruck as when I first saw her fourteen years ago. When I jarred her memory by reminding her of the retreat where we first met, she grew very quiet, looked away and said, "the ribbon on the door". I smiled, and she looked at me for a very long time. She remembered.

Perhaps because our friendship was begun in silence, words did not add or detract from our time together or from the testimony that her spirit was giving me. Love, or God had become so intimately fused with her flesh, it could be seen peeking from every pore. Something tender, something sweet yet with a certain grandeur asserted its greater power and commanded a taller reverence and respect.

Gazing upon my friend in her frail body, I felt the same awe of gazing upon a mountain peak. So this is what becomes of *a feeling of love*, of love consciousness when it is allowed to burgeon. Somehow, out of the deterioration of the mind and the settling of and returning to earth of the body, *the spirit retains its first blush: fresh gurgle of life and glow of radiant wellness*.

My friend's spirit stayed with me long after our visit, its sweetness and love palpable. Somehow, at some point in her labors of love, she had reconnected herself to an original source, which remained undiminished and ready to return to its creator. A quality of sweetness within a sense of consciousness and love is a second way we can describe the power of love consciousness.

Much like Hildegard, Meister Eckert in trinitarian fashion

articulates a third power emanating and pouring from the Holy Spirit through Jesus, "*mit Süßigkeit und Reichtum ohne Maß*" [lxxxv](sweetness and richness without measure) "then the soul flows into itself and out of itself, overflowing itself and over all things through grace with force (*gewaltig*) without a medium back again to its first beginning."[lxxxvi] (*ersten Beginn -Ursprung*) (parenthesis mine).

Both Hildegard and Meister Eckert point to a love and sweetness that is poured forth, from the Urgrund, or Ursprung, that is, primitive beginnings of existence. And our ultimate fulfillment in this life is the eventual return of these love feelings to their source. Julian of Norwich recollects "three kinds of demeanour in our Lord…the third, and that is the blessed demeanour, partly like what it will be in heaven; and that is when through grace we are touched by sweet illuminations of the life of the Spirit, through which we are kept in true faith, hope and love, with contrition and devotion and also with contemplation and every kind of true joys and sweet consolations."[lxxxvii]

Making a return to an original love source brings a palpable sense of permanence, and the third quality of the power of love consciousness and of *a feeling of love*, is the lingering sensation of the experience. More than a memory, the feelings are deeply embodied, and remain as a mark long after the initial love gift.

John of the Cross mentions this lingering quality as that which sets apart a vision which is from God and not from a delusion, "For the effects… are not like those produced by good visions; the former produce aridity of spirit as to communion with God and an inclination to esteem oneself highly, …Neither do the forms of such visions remain impressed upon the soul with the sweetness and brightness of the others; nor do they last, but are quickly effaced from the soul, save when the soul greatly esteems them…[lxxxviii]

Sprung from nature, and back to original being, or *Ursprung*. The feeling of love, when nurtured and attended to brings us to fullness of life, to a life that never leaves us, even if our senses and physical faculties fail. We need only gaze, only recognize that it is an inseparable part of us. How can we picture this power of love consciousness?   Perhaps there is no better way than that of the mystic who answered the question "what is your secret?"

'"Well, my secret if you want to call it that, is not much. It is just sort of…an imagination that comes to me when things aren't just up to the mark. It's come to me since I got sick as a lad, and it comes now often in the day. Whenever I stop to think about it, it seems to me that I have spent my entire life sitting in the place of St. John at the Last Supper."'[lxxxix]

Our head, leaning against the breast of God, is how we come into the world, and is ultimately how we part. A life of love is spent along the way, remembering and living this posture and knowing that we know, that we are one, together with original being.   God is within, within *a feeling of love*, and we are sustained in this tender power forever and always.

Community Paradigms

The Lord calls you back, like a wife forsaken and grieved in spirit, A wife married in youth and then cast off, says your God. For a brief moment I abandoned you, but with great tenderness I will take you back.

- (Isaiah 54: 6,7) *New American Bible*

This excerpt, taken from the Easter Vigil liturgy portends the messianic event. Taken in light of the present rise of feminism and mysticism against a backdrop of languishing intimacy and tattered relationships, we can yearn for the yet to be realized dawning of the end of our abandonment. In the interim, we grope among the ashes of crumbling institutions that once provided stability, intimacy and moral ground; or so it seemed, and now leave us scorned and rejected.

Two such institutions, that of marriage and vowed celibacy, remained a bastion of divine embodiment and fulfillment until the sheer numbers of defections evidenced an apparent absence and burgeoning doubt of the presence of God or God's intrinsic goodness in either one. And as Isaiah suggests, the crisis is a loss of meaning; it is a woman's spirit that grieves; intimacy is that which is mourned.

"The new kind of marriage taking shape in our culture demands much more on an interpersonal level of its partners than marriages did in the past; yet we do not seem to have developed the necessary skills at communication, expressing and receiving feelings, supporting each other's personal growth, building friendships outside the marriage-which long-term modern marriage demands."[xc]

As women have gained a voice, every structure, title, role and moral definition (as defined by males) has been questioned, and when found to be inauthentic, stripped of its authority.

But as if to grant misogyny its final coup; women, instead of originating new models and tenets for living, have out of their own sense of reinforced feminine devaluation adopted and moved into male roles and opportunism. Wives who were once regarded as so much chattel in a marriage, now can possess their own. Housewives who suffered from the lack of recognition and personal resources now have the power but the drain and the emotional strain of a career along with the maintenance of a home and the nurture of family intimacy.

Jean Baker Miller points out the reluctance of women to create conflict; and notices "For women to derive strength from relationships...clearly requires a transformation and restructuring of the nature of relationships"[xci]

Constructive criticism and conflict, that which more than a diatribe offers a remedy or new direction was never more needed than in marriage.

There are three ways in which we idealize or recognize marriage in our current western culture. First is that we grant to two persons the desire to stay with and for each other all of their earthly lives. The second embodies the definitive whole of marriage, and that is consummation. For a marriage to exist at all, there must be regular sexual intercourse, even & specifically, as regards some capacity for a Roman Catholic Annulment , there must be penetration of the penis of the man into the vagina of the woman.[xcii] Lastly, marriage must involve a degree of intimacy and love between the partners which is satisfying to both.

A generation or two ago, it was relatively simple to maintain a marriage, largely because of the reduced expectations placed upon it particularly by and toward women. Another factor was the insistence of external constructs and imperatives that became a model for living rather than any integrity or internal reality. As a child I can remember conversations with friends which intimated whose parents were still sleeping together and whose were not. There was a natural progression in many marital relationships at that time which sacrificed personal satisfaction for the good of a moral or social code. There are many marriages even today that stay together for the sake of the children or other moral/social prescription.

Marriage developed out of male patriarchal systems which paid little regard to personal intimacy or if it did, had no model in order to sustain it. Its establishment insured proper lineage, and nuptial coitus was a duty if nothing else. Once a quality of sexual satisfaction was introduced especially for women, and the context of partnerships shifted to love and intimacy, matrimonial bonds of exclusive and ordered sex could stretch but not contain what requires a new paradigm.

Prevailing marital themes revolve around sex, specifically the form which necessitates male penile penetration. This form, outside of occasional procreative functioning, has a down side however when it is established as a social construct and a repetitive, dominant mode of interaction between the sexes. What is considered natural and sacred in a conceptive scene, can quickly become distorted with any alternate intentionality.

"In a warrior culture, once the sword had been proclaimed mightier than the plow, the soldier more potent than the farmer, a man's penis and his weapon became fused...The penis first became a sword and then a gun and the warrior's ritual of manhood became alternately stroking the penis and the rifle while singing the Marine hymn: 'This is my rifle, this is my gun. This is for business, this is for fun.'...Rape was a privilege of the conquering hero in times of war and a habit hard to break in times of peace..."[xciii]

Like the doctor whose slap of the newborn brings air and life, effecting liberty and consciousness to a bit of divine breath, we dare not think to raise our own hand to an infant otherwise; the same act is sapped of its integrity and vigor by displacing it from original intentionality. Regardless of affection, professionalism, or rank, the person who receives penetration of any sort at the impulse of another whether it be a dental exam or a splinter removal, is vulnerable, and this vulnerability is not mutual.

In kind, every woman who is heterosexually active, in spite of whatever loving overtures may have accompanied her history of intercourse, knows to some degree what rape feels like. Passivity to penetration is something which as human beings we seek to avoid, and males are reflective of this normative behavior in their strong reactions toward homosexual males. Gay men are erroneously believed to engage in anal sex, and this is interpreted to mean that men receive and yield to penetration.

"The gay male threatens other males because he embodies the symbol of woman. Stereotypically, it is assumed that in gay male sexual intercourse one of the partners must be passive and take the woman's role. But the assumption that a man would willingly submit to "womanization" can be a symbolic threat to every other male..."[xciv]

When references to sex become interchangeable with "making love" and physical intimacy, there is another difficulty in being able to distinguish love from sex. We intuit that there is something intimate in coming to know the erotic responses of a person we love, especially if that is revealed in a period of mutual nakedness. Also, there are hints of affection and love if our union occurs with marked gentleness and care, including kisses and caresses. But when we expect these elements to manifest themselves simultaneously, as grafted onto one another, we preclude anything in its singular fullness of experience to compare them to (fulfilling our assumptions); or anything to expand or challenge our experiences of human physical love. Forcing "love" out of a particular action, in this case, that of penetrative sex, is not only counter to how love works, but also stints the growth and possibilities that love holds for the two involved. If love is synonymous with an act in marriage, one only need to fulfill the act. For males, this only reinforces considerable ambiguity.

"We are so easily confused about intimacy. Because we have genitalized so much of our sexual feelings, intimacy and sex seem to be one and the same. Thus, if we are heterosexual, we fear intimacy with other men because it seems to imply genital expression. And deep emotional intimacy with women threatens our masculinity, because we learned our first lessons about manhood by the process of breaking the erotic bonding with a woman, our mother."[xcv]

Indeed, we know that the ability to be vulnerable is at the core of genuine love and intimacy, and because of the vulnerability that is offered each time a man inserts his penis into the vagina of a woman, it is hard to doubt that this does in fact offer instant intimacy to men. In the cases where women are not able to erotically or orgasmically participate, men are also offered unconditional tenderness and affection. It is interesting to view male sexuality from the perspective that, as a gender and in their patriarchal structures they have as a group and as an ideology been in aggressive pursuit and protection of intimacy by the natural means they possess.

For women, there is a deep and far-reaching downside to contemporary models for marriage. Because sex does not equal love, the toll of intimacy taken but not usually returned increases with age. Anger and resentment surface as conditions of what Stephen Covey might call "too many withdrawals and not enough deposits".[xcvi] It is small wonder perhaps, when a woman in her later years is not valued or prized in our society. Once sexual attractiveness is deemed wanting by our cultures' standards, the terms applied to aging femininity seem to reflect the gamut of an embittered gender "crone...matriarch, harridan, hag, battle-axe and old bag...

Social attitudes to growing older and the emphasis on women being attractive and young may in themselves impose on us or exacerbate an existing sense of loss at the time of the menopause. This feeling of losing something is the basis on which women evaluate themselves in self-deprecating and derogatory terms. We see ourselves as if reflected in a distorting mirror erected by society."[xcvii]

Sexual activity is often enhanced or attributed to alcoholic influences, so that I was entertained to find that in German, the word *Rausch* for inebriation, can be combined with the word *Zeit*, or time, and used to mean "mating season". The imbalance of the fertile years, a time of coupling and multiplying, which for a male is a step toward good health, and for women, a prescription for depression, can perhaps be attributed to a time in a woman's life when she is not only intoxicated by the newness of pleasure but subdued as well by the unegalitarian and demanding pressures of our marriage symbol. In adolescence, a time of peak sexual attractiveness and preoccupation,

"...[women] undergo a gradual change in which they lose

their feisty spirit, courage, and willingness to speak out-qualities they had known in girlhood. Around this time their truth becomes silenced, held back. They become afraid of conflict with males, because they know on some level that males hold the power. They become-perhaps forever-good little girls, settling into the cliches and limits imposed on their gender."[xcviii]

Only one third of women are able to orgasm to the same degree of frequency that their male partners enjoy. Given the choice, women do not come to pleasure by means of deep penetration when masturbating. Rape, and the fear of rape are not moments of sexual intimacy; and women are daily on the defensive for them. In rape, over and above other crimes of power and passion, it is purely the violation, the willful probing of one's body by another that fosters the unique horror and the risk. Compounding these elements of sexual experience women fear pregnancy during normal intercourse which affects their psychological comfort and ease of enjoyment; and in some cases where there are health risks to conception, even death. Physical closeness which as a prerequisite exacts the capitulation of the feminine body may very likely be at the root of rape fantasies that consume the same women who enjoy them with guilt; and serve to fuel pornography and male aggression.

For males, there is the fear of impotence, and feelings of being "engulfed" by the vagina. Both men and women have numerous concerns over health and the change within a relationship that sex brings. Instead of genuine freedom, penetrative sex threatens untold attachments including unwanted children, disease, and even death.

Most married couples do not know what is pleasing to their partner in their coming together for genital sexuality, except perhaps for a dim sense of what is or is not "working" in the aim of orgasm for each other.

This cannot be called intimacy, and certainly not love. Though these individuals it can be said for the most part enjoy each other and this mutual activity usually does carry with it an exclusive or limited license of participation, it is amazing nonetheless how our prevaling dialogue of sexuality interchangeably inserts "physical intimacy", "intimacy", "physical love", and "love making" when intending sex.

Our language may betray our true longings. Instead of love, however, we are led into arrangements in which there is not necessarily acceptance of every portion of our partner's body. Because sex as we now know it involves technique, skill, fantasies and private preferences, we may spend a lifetime and not be kissed and reverenced over every inch of our bodies. Naked yet incomplete, sex breaks into portions the periphery of a significant other toward the accomplishment of a goal. That goal is not necessarily love.

The procreative posture when mimicked as the mode of intimacy in marriage has the advantage of being readily duplicated and enforced. Because it replicates a natural form of congress, when it is coupled with embracing and kissing, it can easily be adapted to feel more natural and affectionate than more explicit erotic forms of pleasure, such as oral or anal sex, or mutual petting. Everyone knows how to do it, and it is easy to learn.

All of this is not to imply that recreative penetrative sex ought to be verboten in a new paradigm. Personal choice and freedom of spirit is the central issue for a new vision. The core or context of physical intimacy, and not what would be incidental or digressive displays of affection, play or eroticism are what set the overall tone of mutuality and intimacy. Keeping traditional intercourse as the norm and requirement is a detriment however, to self-sustaining love relationships. The current model requires only external conformity and not an internal openness in the impetus to love. We can break into and out of new models.

"...our embodiment is so thoroughly historical, that we must be ever-wary of assertions that any particular cultural mediation of the body's meaning is a 'given' of nature and of human fate. Biology is not destiny. Neither is freedom disincarnate."[xcix]

A hurdle is created when the traditional form of sexual interaction loses strength, and a couple then must consider settling into a routine, becoming mostly or entirely celibate or seeking professional forms of assistance by way of couseling, instructional videos and literature. The latter can seem complicated or unnatural, since they offer various sexual or nonsexual techniques which must be learned and developed in order to restart an erotic spark, and are not readily available except for those who are humble or courageous enough, or economically capable to search them out.

A good marriage can evolve into an elite category of those who read the self help books and can afford to attend weekends or pay babysitters, therapists etc. A good marriage then is assimilated as being a commodity just like having a large home, two cars, and doing better than just keeping up with many of the neighbors. Sophistication is applicable even to those who may not have exerted a great deal of effort in their relationships, so that a myth of "success" is mutual between couples instead of humble love and intimacy.

No one has definitively articulated what a "good marriage" is. The only rule is that it somehow is lasting, though no one knows how long is lasting enough. The claim among many couples is that they have a good marriage, and this is prior to an ensuing divorce; and a divorce can occur at any time during a good marriage, early on or fifty years into the relationship.

What remains are only questions: What really is a good marriage? How do we know if a marriage is long lasting? Does marriage connote a success that a single or divorced person is lacking? Does the state of marriage carry extra love and intimacy that a single individual cannot contain in their lifestyle?

Wherever we decide to look, the answers are not to be found in a definitive way in the Christian church. Though there is evidence that a spiritual union in which there is mutual meditation and ritual between a couple seems to participate in longevity and quality of relationship, the component of spiritual awareness is one that is required and understood only in the tender model. It is extraneous and difficult however in the sexual paradigm, where the ideal is expressed in terms of the Pauline extract; marriage is realized as just like that relationship between Christ and the church.

"...[the author probably not Paul] takes a symbol of the eschatological union of Christ and the Church, which is actually antithetical to human marriage and sexuality, and tries to impose it inappropriately on human marriage in order to counteract the tendencies of the early Church to dissolve marriage into eschatalogical equality between celibate women and men. The author is caught midway between the Pauline eschatalogical vision of the Church and the reactionary direction of the household codes, which try to return the Christian Church to the models of historical patriarchy. The result is a contradiction that, nevertheless, for two thousand years has been preached to Christian couples as though it were a possible model of real marriage."[c]

A friend once shared her amazement when she and her husband discovered that they communicated differently in an embrace. Prompted by something they saw in a video, they began to exchange what they felt and preferred in an embrace and were astonished at the new understanding they acquired after several years of marriage.

In fact, such probing into the intentionality of physical intimacy is a large step forward for a relationship that is sex centered. But on the scale of tender intimacy and love making, it is but a baby step, toward loving awareness and intensely powerful ecstasy. Waves, not ripples of intimacy are what two persons may embark upon if the strong societal currents of genital action are circumvented.

These tides are extremely strong. There is enormous pressure in our society to be sexually active, and if sexually active, satisfied as well. Somehow, there prevails a double standard which states that even though conventional sex is no longer seen as procreation only or even primarily, it is still one of the "facts of life". Sex in marriage is promulgated as something God created for marital intimacy instead of the social construct which we know and believe it to be.

It may be time to reconsider an act involving penetration which as symbol of relationship may lay vulnerable and inferior an entire gender along with its imitators. To create life, penile insertion is necessary. But the "facts" extend this behavior like a cloak to the entirety of associations between the genders.

A procreative stance, as something that is essential and God ordained, somehow creeps into everyday lives in marriage, and is not reserved for those rare moments when a new life is urged forth from a couples' communion. In spite of inconsistencies, genital coupling is never questioned as occupying the central role in any intimate relationship.

Because penetrative sex is at the core of intimacy between the genders, it also sits symbolically at a pivotal point in the conflicts arising from feminist consciousness. The same anthropomorphic stance that places man at the intentional focus of nature and the universe, usurps the nature of procreation for personal gain. Ecofeminism upholds the importance of shifting from a power over nature stance to one that is aware of being nature oneself. Elizabeth Johnson urges "a new vision...The precise point has been to overcome sexist disparagement of the female in the three basic relationships of human beings among each other, with the earth, and with God, and thereby to serve the future of life itself."[ci]

Sandra Schneiders notes,

"Feminist spirituality is the reclaiming by women of the reality and power designated by the term 'spirit' and the effort to reintegrate spirit and body, heaven and earth, culture and nature, eternity and time, public and private, political and personal, in short, all those hierarchized dichotomous dualisms whose root is the split between spirit and body and whose primary incarnation is the split between male and female."[cii]

Consequently, to alter the most basic way a man and a woman come together in primary intimacy is to realign more than one relationship. But the answer does not lie in the ingestion of a male hormone in order to increase a woman's aggressive sexual behavior and fantasies, as recommended by a gynecologist on a public television program. The answer is also not in the invention of a new posture of sexual intercourse as I will describe later, although this is a wonderful step toward leveling the playing field for the sake of women and increasing the possibilities of sexual enhancement for both male and female.

Instead of one more attempt which bolsters the male experience as normative, and apart from an additional technique for social marketing, we require a model of lovemaking that is entirely natural, and intrinsically love. This model in turn must become the definitive embodiment of a relationship of tender love. It must be easily understood, and it must be regarded as "better" in total physical, emotional and spiritual satisfaction and enjoyment.

As we regard the players in our arbitrary arrangements of codes and customs it is possible to cast the male role in its dominance and aggression with that of the power which acts upon nature, and opposed to the power of being and nature. This is similar to Scilla Elworthy's comparison of the "power over" to what she terms "hara power".

Thus the body may receive gratification, but the rest of the person remains distanced.

The alternative would be an approach in which the whole person - mind, body and spirit - is present in sex, and in which the body again becomes central to our daily lives in every sense, not simply tucked away and ignored except when we want gratification. Scilla suggests differences in a hara approach to lovemaking:

"We do not much mind whether lovemaking includes orgasm or not; it is the closeness that matters.

Lovemaking is not a means to something, it is an end in itself.

I want to become one with you, not remain as two; I want to move into the act so deeply that the actor is no more."[ciii]

But as discussed in the mystical chapter there is a third power, which must be brought to bear in order to maintain the necessary salubrious harmony.

The work of George Ivanovitch Gurdjieff as articulated by Peter Brooks recognizes in our everyday conception of quality, a state of higher energy or "presence", which when lacking, leaves us to agitate and take sides in the battle of humanism over science; more primally, the importance of spirit over matter and man over woman...

"The transformation of a human being only begins when the sources in the body, ...cease to produce spasmodic and erratic bursts of energy and begin to function harmoniously together.

Then, for the first time, a new quality appears, which Gurdjieff calls "presence". As the intensity of presence rises, the matrix of our reactions and desires, which we call the ego, gradually becomes elastic and transparent, and in the center of our automatic structure of behavior a new space is formed in which a true individuality can arise."[civ]

One woman shared her experience of transformation after an evening of tender lovemaking,

Earlier, while we were walking in the park after dark, I was startled by a sudden rustle. He tried to comfort me by saying that I never needed to be afraid if he was there. It was a naive, macho remark, and I was annoyed by the childish invitation to trust in something other than my own experience.

That night on my bed, we tried it. That is, we made love without arousing each other, by trying to kiss the love consciousness in each other...I was amazed that I could sense his thoughts before he spoke them. Encountering his naked masculinity fresh and whole, a desire for his protection filled me even though I did not have any need to be protected. He then voiced his part in that very longing, now in stark contrast to our earlier stroll.

While at my breast, a similar event; he said, "this might sound strange, but I almost wish you were lactating...I could stay here all night long..." Again he spoke my being.

The higher energies of consciousness require an equal level or burst of energy to maintain their frequencies. Without the regular input of presence into our embodied intimacy, our view of the other gender dries up. Given regular jolts of sex, the other is partitioned and exaggerated by their organs and endowments. Our approach to living is cloaked and guided with a like analysis, the pieces over the whole, the bang for the buck, seduction preemptive of stewardship, and stimulation versus nurture.

The quality of presence increases parallel with the cognition of God or the sacred. When we draw ourselves to respond to our lover as a vessel carrying us into the kiss of the Holy, then and only then do we fully actualize the ecstatic groans of our spirit. Satisfaction takes place for the first time. We are irrevocably altered, mended. We understand many things, above all as Beatrice Bruteau notes, that there must be three:

"Remember that this kind of loving is not admiring or desiring or enjoying. It's giving yourself to the other in union with the other's own subjectivity. So if the other's own subjectivity is engaged in loving a third party, your act of loving has to be joining in this.

Since the whole nature of a Divine Person is love, the First Lover is bound to find that what the subjectivity of the Beloved is doing is loving, and so the First Lover's love is realized only when joined to the Second Lover's act of loving the Third Person."[cv]

Ecstatic union resultant of overwhelming love of body, mind and spirit fulfills our requisites.

As an adolescent and through adulthood, I can remember the numerous gropings in physical intimacy with men, none of which felt natural or tender. But at least initially, I was being inducted into another world, and I felt as though I was the one that needed to learn. One fellow, after I decided to retreat the lines of our sexual petting, received a tender embrace from me and smirked. I needed to make up my mind, he said, with complete authority. Slowly I was being indoctrinated into a for-sex-only society.

And the countless styles of french kissing; none of them felt right, none of them moved me deeply, and yet I would relish the fantasies that replayed them over and over erotically in my mind. The next kiss then became more and more instantaneously erotic, and after a while there was only one thing on each of our minds.

There was one man with a wonderful style, but it was not natural, though the technique was smooth. If I exclaimed any feelings while we were aroused and naked, if I tried to gaze at him with love, he was annoyed by the distraction. He had to keep his erection, after all; that was hard work.

It is my conviction that women and men who know the difference between what it means to be tender and what it means to be sexual must teach that difference. Our entire world and its happiness depend upon it. If we are to move with integrity toward a more fulfilling life and a new paradigm for physical lovemaking and intimacy, it must look something like this:

Sit facing each other in a comfortable position, close

together. Place your left hand over your partner's heart, letting it extend slightly over her left breast. Allow your partner to place her left hand over your heart. Now place your right hand on top of her left which is positioned over your heart. Let your partner place her right hand on top of your left which is positioned over her heart.

"Now stare deeply, directly into the eyes - those beautiful eyes that are true windows to the soul. Continue to become lost in the eyes, those wonderful eyes through which love is automatically communicated. Become lost in the eyes which sparkle with energy and glisten with emotion. Become aware of your heartbeat and your partner's heartbeat. Feel the breathing, breathing each free and gentle and easy breath together. You are now sharing the very essence of life with each breath that you take, breathing in the same air.

You are exchanging energy in the very air that you breathe...You are loving your partner with pure positive thought energy, touching and stroking your partner mentally...You are becoming a channel of flowing energy. You can feel the tingling energy flowing from your body to your partner's body and back again...Tingling energy is flowing through your body to your partner from your partner back into you...

You are becoming lost in the experience now - just perceiving and flowing, flowing waves of energy from one body to the other...You can feel that glowing, eager sexual arousal, that indescribable kind of anticipation. And you may notice an unusual peacefulness along with your arousal. But there's a quickening of the spirit and a tingling of the genitals. Just allow yourself to become lost in the free-flowing intensity of the experience. Let the intimacy build until it takes you to new heights of ecstasy and new levels of love."[cvi]

Paul Pearsal describes a posture of the future, in which two lovers face each other with their legs intertwined. The left leg of one partner bends and is placed over the right leg of the other, while the right leg is underneath the other's left leg, wrapping itself about their back. In this position, the arms are free. The underside of the man's penis can rest against the clitoris of the woman, maximizing the stimulation of each one's most pleasurable areas.

"You have learned about a new sexual system. You know that there is no reason to limit yourself to the old views of sex that emphasized penetration, thrusting, orgasm, timing, energy release, and ejaculation. To learn more about this, you may want to try a posture that emphasizes the new sexual system, one that stresses closeness, time-free interaction, pays no attention to erection, penetration, ejaculation, or orgasm, but allows for intense and mutual psychasm...."[cvii]

The above passages superimportantly level the playing field between a man and a woman. When we look again at the opening passage from Isaiah, we notice that to replace "wife" with "husband" leaves the lines feeling less poignant, and missing the same ardent pathos that a woman emits in the same circumstances. Marriage must never be an institution which constructs, solidifies and normalizes the helpless dependancy of either a man or a woman. Such a paradigm can only result in something that is spiritually crippling, and emotionally unsustainable.

Deeply Loving Friendships

'If it happens that a disciple comes to see his master less and less, but remembers him more and more at home, what does this signify?' ' It is better', replied the master, 'for someone to be absent from his master and remember him than to be present with him all day yet not be touched by his love.'

Nizam Ad-Din Awliya

An experience of deep love with limerance, and with spiritual reverance as its foundation, has been a part of the human make up since the beginning of time, since the Garden of Eden. In nature, it is to experience a personal caress where we only sought the comfort and nurture of wilderness. When we open and uncover the consciousness of Divine love in our tendermost center, the physical representations of Divinity matter less and less, while we remember more and more. The hallmark of mystical union is the limerance of Divine presence, everywhere.

While the spiritual relationship between master and disciple has been preserved in most cultures as a non sexual paradigm of relationship, this has also been isolated as such from our ordinary human friendships. The deep love of a soul sharing relationship has been left unexplored, as part and parcel of a spiritual, physical and emotional split.

Yet the ability to establish a spiritually tender bond is pivotal to not only an understanding of mystical union, but also to a retrieval of fullness of love and the total completeness which has been ours promised from the dawn of life.

Deep, undifferentiated longing for we know-not-what, it is also a tap root for "inner strength". We draw and groan and cry from it when a trauma or crisis has eradicated all that once supported our ego strength and fragile sense of self. It is where love's consciousness returns to refound our truth. It is the signature of God, and tumultuously, birth. The power it emanates is one which dominates and suspends the power of being or nature and the power which is set against nature.

Appearing as love, wind, fire, water and birth, these are similar manifestations of the power of love's consciousness. It is a struggle to name this power, except to hail it as Yahweh (I am who am). Cleansing, purifying, restorative, and life renewing, brought together in a conduit which bent in tender contact to the original power of being and nature sets all of creation in harmony. In symbol as well as form, love's language is composed with eloquence as "fire of passion", overflowing and gushing, "breath" and "warmth", and we often are said to be "reborn", in love and spirit into our truest selves.

"In the beginning was the word..." This first passage from the gospel of John, notes Gurdjieff, recalls a time when there was not yet a form of language or of words. We could therefore suggest, that in the beginning was the sound,[cviii] and the harmonic creation integral to his philosophy. Similarly, in a context in which there are no sounds or vibrations without breath and the movement of air, we can paraphrase John, "In the beginning was the word, he who was borne of wind..."

Daily we fashion lifestyles which combat the elements, only to discover that all of our efficiency is halted in a moment of storm, water, fire and wind. In the midst even, of destruction, sorrow and despair we may experience an influx of consciousness; in rebirth, beauty, and joy in suffering. Like rain which instantaneously bursts lush foliage forth in a desert, enormous birthing surrounds and awaits these elements.

Once in a workshop on death and dying, I remember the woman who was leading the discussion describe dying as one more portal through which we inevitably pass, like birth. Her own life after a period of time in hospice work became in her words, "sweeter and more tender". Especially in death, where wind, warmth and moisture are forever released, it is only the promise of love's consciousness that may suspend and contain its own resurrection. We have the potentiality of housing Divine consciousness, so that when our vessels are no more, love may become home and enclosure to our souls.

Impregnated we experience and embody the heat, the moisture, and breathe life and love. The common identifier for all of these most elemental points of existence is that they cannot be self-contained. Ironically, though they are unattainable, intimately we are joined and in harmony with each. Only, we need to see that it is so.

But in essence, the power which sets itself against nature interrupts the power of being. The same is true of the power of love consciousness. This has the capacity to nullify the power which sets itself against nature. Though they are all equal, there is a three tiered echelon of which one power may suspend the other.

So that, even when there is death and destruction, suffering and loss, the palpable beauty of the experience, even the joy, become attainable, when love's consciousness intrudes upon the aggresive power acting against being and nature. "Joy is strength", I believe is attributed to Mother Teresa. Well, then true strength is of the same channel as joy. Our inner strength touched with love's consciousness becomes the light and love, the joy which permeates and powers our life.

In practical terms, say that someone has been tenderly touched by the care and concern of someone else. Perhaps that someone else is a woman. Then the first person has had their elemental longings activated and is becoming filled with thoughts of the woman. In a fantasy, the individual finds themselves at the woman's breast. Alarmed, the person then thinks that, because of cultural and social interpretations, this must be something sexual. Then there are decisions to be made, especially if the person is a married male, or if they are a woman. The latter might seriously feel threatened by the implications that she is a lesbian or besexual. Neither is true, in and of itself.

In actuality, the imagined event, with the conscious freedom and permission of the beloved woman can be practiced with the original tender conveyance or consciousness of love in the moment, without accoutrements, or, no movement forward or progression. If consciousness is slowed or even stopped, a different interpretation might be discovered. Or, the person touched by love could call to mind the God within the beloved woman at that moment, until eroticism is suspended, and love is recovered. There was never anything to fear or risk in the first place.

But I am not implying here that there is no such thing as homosexuality. That would be insulting and simplistic to those who have sincerely struggled and embraced not only the posture but the lifestyle as well. Many persons however, having read my drafts of these chapters have been able to admit for the first time that they have enjoyed deep love for someone of the same sex and have felt enabled and liberated as never before. Without a doubt, perhaps in addition to an understanding of something that is homosexual, there is a truth which needs to be spoken, so that the love within the human spirit may be liberated in a way that is not currently possible in our culture.

God is love, and in love there is no male or female. Liberation is freedom, the wilderness that cannot be self contained, that which is God consciousness, joined to our fabric in our mother's womb. We might commit ourselves to a hetero or homosexual lifestyle and continue to fall in love. Do we cut off these feelings as abnormal? Do we refuse to act on these longings and genuine care? Absolutely not.

The failure of the current thinking about long term commitments is that it attempts to self -contain love, which is wild and un-self-containable. It just isn't possible in any authentic way to make love exclusive. Divorce also cannot separate a familial bond like that formed among mothers and fathers and children. We place enormously false expectations as a culture in either direction. More responsibility can only be placed where there is the hope of some control, where it may in fact be actualized in the type of lifestyle chosen, especially when children are in the plan.

As a culture we must recognise the need for families to be supported even in divorce, that there is no such thing as a "broken" family. The attempt, moreover, to break the familial bond along with the sexual or matrimonial separation is the crux of the stress in todays culture. The social paradigm we have is that of a conditional relationship based upon specified acts of closeness within the marriage, instead of an unconditional relationship of nurture and care which would continue even if the sexual attachments weaken, especially when children have extended the forms of commitment.

The focal point becomes the relationship between the parents instead of the relationships with and among the children. In my experience, for example, the parent that attempts to maintain family get togethers is often accused of trying to hang on to the marriage instead of the family, and is thereby forced to give up attempts to do so. What our assumptions about marriage and family lead to in these instances is only intense negativity, stigma and destruction, and not creativity and the many possibilities of love that surround the separated parent family. The challenge remains for us to found creative opportunities of healing and reverancing, supporting and ritualizing as a community the strain of changes in a family makeup just as we do in the instance of a death or illness.

We must also be honest and real in opening up a sexual relationship to the supportive possibilities that other loves are in our future. Genuine love is far too expansive to be enclosed in a paradigm for marriage today. We are only too ready to concede that in order to eliminate a body/spirit split in thinking, we must move forward in the awareness that love is fully physical in its longings and not merely sexual. And if we love fully, we must open ourselves to physical intimacy as well as care for the spiritual and emotional well being of our close friend. Otherwise, the trap of our birthright of original sin remains, never to allow the light of divine consciousness completion and transformation of our horizon.

"It has long been noted that the process of spiritual awakening and growth is associated with periods of rising sexual passion". Gerald May notes what appears to be a paradox within spiritual relationships, or any relationship which becomes touched by love's tender consciousness. Because even though we might attempt an erotic sexual encounter, "it is never finally satisfying because it always represents a side-tracking of one's primary longing." May correctly describes the best most holy form of sexual communion as a "celebration" and goes on to make an important distinction " celebrations of God's creation and searching for deeper relationship *with* God are not quite the same thing."[cix]

We have learned to lump all of our longings into one basket of erotic maneuvering. In the case of a love relationship then, we are forced to choose either sexual closeness with a sacrificed satisfaction of longing or distant, non physically intimate expressions of love. With whatever noble intentions we desperately gather to assuage our painful separation, we erect a dam of humble submition to the unruliness of our aroused passion.

But in fact, God never meant for us to suffer this alienation from our true longing in its Divine source within our selves or within a spiritual friend. Unlike sex, tender lovemaking actually can be the same thing as our search for deeper relationship with God. So our bodies are not trying to trick us, and God is not cruel. Our bodies are aroused in raw undifferentiated longing that "knows that it knows " it may find fulfillment in another spiritual person. We seriously lack a model and a map.

One obstacle is the way we have become accustomed to

viewing our bodies. We see our embodiment as something that wraps and contains our spirits, in a way that doesn't allow anything to escape, like earthen vessels, until we pass from this life, our bodies die, and we are able to leave our earthly prisons and become one with God. This is the standard which has been passed down through a Judeo Christian tradition. In this case, sex is a matter of neat fitting between two clay cups, in a small portion of which little grooves and pieces were made for one another. The insides never necesarily need or can spill over, but this is our only refuge from hopeless exile. And with such an image, this is the best we can hope for.

But the human form is much more like a weave. Through all of the pores, orifices, each of the five senses, we emit, emot, communicate, warm and moisten. Much, much more is really passing through than is ever really contained. Looking at it this way, it seems to miss the big picture if we were to attempt to couple a small portion of the entire knit of humanity. Better to oh so simply, allow these individuals to bring to proximity the entirety of their raw, undifferentiated longing and wait; letting them breathe and surrender and cohere as one mesh together.

Where we prefer the power to act upon nature, this is all too elusive and unquantifiable. Once in a meeting with a woman who instructed sacred dance to adolescents, I asked her what guidelines she required of the students in order to conform to what might be legitimately considered sacred motion and movement. This was prompted by my own picture of a room full of teenagers who might revel much more in rebellion and profanity than in an establishment protected and promulgated view of the Holy. Her response startled me. None, she said, and explained that the young adults found sacred movement and dance to come very naturally.

The result is the realization that while sex and dance is a social construct, i.e. the power to act upon nature, sacred expression is something that comes to us innately and directly. No one leads! There are no predetermined acts or scripts. We move to whatever spirit is diffused through the openings of our bodies.

Place the power of love's consciousness within a relationship and eroticism is suspended. Raw undifferentiated longing and surrender are all that remain. In Sufism, "In the most extreme formulation, the disciple was to be to the master like a corpse in the hands of a corpse-washer...the relationship between the two was indicated by the term *irada*, meaning longing or desire. The disciple is called the *murid*, or one who desires, while the master is the *murad*, or the one who is desired."[cx]

Nothing is cut and dried, black and white or dualistic. Through our "mesh" we behold both the physical and spiritual. A new paradigm for deeply loving friendships is a map more in contradistinction from the typically sexual bond. Two persons, instead of being an item, sitting next to each other, holding hands when others are present, open outward instead. The exclusive nature of two persons who belong to each other vaporizes. Rather, they move in and out, one from the other. Because the experience of love is not eroticized, and is therefore not explicitly found in physical contact, no programs, expectations, or jealousy is present, since one does not belong to the private joys and pleasures of the other's body.

Yet it does not resemble the average close friendship either. The power of love consciousness suspends eroticism, as we have seen in the case with the tantric couple, but unlike most close friends, it risks sexual involvement nonetheless, going farther than it ever thought possible without the derailment of passions running willfully on their own. What was once thought only to be suspiciously sexual in subconscious intent, love's tender consciousness is now opened up, and we arrive at a certainty and knowing, in spite of how this consciousness remains very much mixed into our erotic sexuality.

"God grant that I may be able to understand this, and even more that I may be able to describe it, for I am not sure that I know when love is spiritual and when there is sensuality mingled with it, or how to begin speaking about it." St Theresa of Avila goes on to describe how someone immersed in love's consciousness is less attached to material and physical pleasure yet enjoys it more.

"Do you suppose that such persons will love none and delight in none save God? No; they will love others much more than they did, with a more genuine love, with greater passion with a love which brings more profit; that in a word, is what love really is...do you ask again, by what they are attracted if they do not love things they see? They do love what they see and they are greatly attracted by what they hear; but the things which they see are everlasting. If they love anyone they immediately look right beyond the body, fix their eyes on the soul and see what there is to be loved in that."[cxi]

When two can abide in the contemplation not of the periphery or hull of a person but pass through the living weave with a vision and love of the soul, the relationship is elevated to something extraordinary. It is unfortunately, however, a love that is counter to the prevailing paradigms.

"Invariably this occurs among priests and men and women religious in their sixties and seventies. They have finally found someone with whom they can be warm and intimate in non-genital ways. In other words, they have experienced sexual intimacy, possibly for the first time. Yet they do not feel free to share their relationships with those among whom they live. When I ask if they are doing anything to violate their vows or promises, or if they are abusing the relationship in any way, they always say with some degree of surprise, "Well, no!" "Well, why can't you share the good news of your relationship with your confreres?," I ask. "They wouldn't understand," is the response I continually hear."[cxii]

The religious celibate lifestyle, present in all traditions to some degree, is one which uniquely fosters tender love. But the gift is present within a strange paradox, made difficult only by what our sexual expectations and conditioning have risen to become.

"In their avoidance of personal contact, repressed persons are, in fact, unchaste. They are unable to fulfill the fundamental demand of chastity: unconditional reverance for life, the whole of life, including genital feelings. People who avoid personal relations by repressing feelings separate tenderness (affectivity) from the whole of life. Infatuated people never do so, for the integrating power of eros will not permit such a separation."[cxiii]

In this paragraph Tyrrell equates tender feelings with genital feelings or eros. If we take his meaning in the broader context of sexuality which he intends, then the whole of our celibate or chaste interactions are to some degree repressed. And our primary stance in life is celibacy, when we consider that even if sexually active, only one person generally out of our whole sphere of intimate contacts receives genital attention.

The most popular confession I receive when friends read my work is that in their past, they have fallen in love with someone of the same sex, and now feel the freedom to declare these feelings openly. Often, they were rebuffed from pursuing a reverential relationship by the other party under the guise of impropriety.

Repeatedly, it is reinforced that on the one hand, we are encouraged to love one another; on the other, falling in love is equated with sexual striving and our feelings must be repressed for fear of betraying the "genital" source of our love; on yet another that repression is not good, healthy or viable as an alternative.

We can particularly detect a polarization of sexual attitudes in the contemporary disdain of celibacy as a chosen life option. Remarkably, this is ignored by celibate religious institutions as a whole, while they at the same time struggle with a loss of meaning and vocations to their lifestyle.

In a secular text by Sally Cline the truth of the disparity of value toward celibacy exists over and against even unusual sexual behavior. So that,

"Adultery, cuckolding, nymphomania, priapism, satyriasis, sodomy and whoring are accepted as either natural or reasonable. Even homosexuality, lesbianism, and sado-masochism, once defined as abnormal, are tolerated on the grounds that at least they involve genital activity... "

After detailing the material content of the pornography industry (which she notes is the largest media category) she concludes,

"As far as 'sex' goes, anything goes, except not going along with the notion at all. Today it is celibacy rather than assault which is viewed as indecent."[cxiv]

Probably these mixed messages are due to the influence of

the male approach to sexuality and intimacy, particularly that of the repressed male. Therefore, at the core of our current paradigm, is a very masculine experience. Crosby admits,

"Men, it seems, can easily confuse the need for sexual intimacy with their sexual needs and desires. Thus men often conflate intimacy with sexual contact(s)."[cxv]

This conflation is precisely what must go in order to form a new paradigm. It is the reason why all of our attempts at sexual freedom and intimacy have backfired. We suffered enormously under a mental and moral structure which saw the body and especially the genitals as something to overcome and control. Now in our courageous efforts to discard and heal past debilitations from feelings of shame and guilt our cups are running over with new experiences and freedom and new paths of destruction. But in the loss of any advancement of intimacy or values that might be noble or profound, many are now eager to turn back the clock.

Instead, the dregs at the bottom of the cup, left over from the old perspectives toward intimacy are what must be dealt with. In terms of the three powers, we are in an eternal ping pong match of the power of being and nature and the power which acts upon nature. Sex as the social construct is a power which acts against nature, yet as the power of procreation is part of our being and nature. When two bodies come into extended contact, the power of love's longing is activated, but the power of sex keeps suspending it. So love's longing and fulfillment is glimpsed, but then averted. Therefore we have two conflicting traditions that say sex is lovemaking, and at the same time that sex is pleasure seeking.

Now when we experience the influx of love's consciousness, in ways large and small, we know that this suspends the power of sex as a construct. Therefore, an entire tradition establishes sex as evil and a distraction from the spiritual, and God and spirituality as not bodily connected.

Continually, we have been missing the point. It is not that sex is evil. It is also not true that spirituality exists apart from our bodies. What we must accomplish, the missing piece we need to replace, is the bringing together of the power of love's consciousness to the power of being and nature. In other words, do you pray and meditate in the arms of a beloved? Or do you need to go apart to pray? In our current paradigm you have to go apart. In our new paradigm, you become apart of one another's weave.

A new paradigm would incorporate something like this,

"You can do this meditation together with your partner, as a couple, by sitting back to back with your spines in contact over their whole length. This practice will help eliminate fears in your relationship and open deeper communication. At the end of the session push your backs firmly together for a minute or so. Do this, and nothing will come between you!"[cxvi]

How might a religious community, or close friends see their friendship transformed with such a routine? The possibilities are endless, once there is a nongenital and unconditional commitment. Because of the relaxation and peaceful consciousness that prayerful touch brings about, the risks are quickly perceived as unsubstantiated. More, just knowing that sexual satisfaction is not the source or end of our physical longing is in itself a help toward easing our sexual tensions and concerns.

The intimacy and grounded sense of community that tender touch provides also introduces a profound value and strengthens integrity and charity. It is the longing for signs of deeper comforts and truths that support a concept of religious life and community in a culture. O'Murchu regards these individuals as "liminal", or inspiring to the culture at large in so far as it seeks such inspiration.

"There seems to prevail in human culture a tendency to embody in a radical and profound way the values we cherish most deeply...It projects onto these liminal groups its deepest hopes, dreams, and aspirations, and requests the liminal person or group to embody and articulate for society at large the deepest values the society holds sacred."[cxvii]

The disdain in which celibacy is currently held in our culture is possibly reflected in the dismantling of Roman Catholic religious communities today. A view of celibacy as a lifestyle devoid of physical intimacy and genital sex smacks of hipocrisy, psychosexual unhealth (repression) with an inability to comprehend the human condition, and an archaic (in its assumed superfluousness) self negation.

The shift in values in our society from celibacy to physical intimacy is what in turn burgeoned forth this book. In the early nineties, while preparing to profess my own religious vows privately, a friend and spiritual director assigned me the task of researching my own concept of celibacy, since this was the cornerstone of the vow. Feeling my own resistance to doing this I realized that she was right. At that point as I shared freely with friends about what I was about to do I received very limited support, and males in particular were unaccepting and seemed even threatened by anything which promoted celibacy.

The confrontations of my friends challenged me to explore deeper into what I was trying to say. I wondered if the language itself was no longer appropriate and conjured the wrong, repressed and unhealthy images of a time gone by. Finally, after enormous soul searching and entering the depths of my sexual, maternal and mystical experiences, the root of what I began to regard as something "tender" began to take shape.

A vow called tenderness opened new possibilities and horizons for me and became an inspiration to friends. Unlike a standard religious celibacy, this was a vow that I could reach and work at with vitality. It also did not pretend to prune all sexual urgings regardless of the possible good these desires might hold. Instead, the physical freedom that a new understanding ushered forth was breathtaking in its import and sacred grandeur.

It seemed to echo the sentiments of religious celibate Francis Rothleuber, when she muses, "what if a whole community of Sisters, what if each one, every woman, was encouraged and free to experience the full vitality of being a woman? Think of the wail and cry all the way to Rome and back.

Would it really be a scandal if we all understood that our sexual energy is a share in God Energy? What a center of life we would become with exploding, creative compassion and freedom. New music, new ways of educating, of healing. It's exciting to think about."[cxviii]

Sexual energy in its broadest sense truly is a share in God

energy. Sifted from its limiting jargon and context of genital arousal, more than a share, it becomes the whole pie. But how to break out of the prison of intimacy we find ourselves in is not easy, though it certainly is simple. Without structures, models, experience, tradition, the possibilities of deep, lasting love remain in frustration.

We are stuck. Longing with love, we lean toward the hope of a love that seeks our liberation and surrender. But the models for these tender intercourses are not only scarce, but they are not talking. Great love hovers, perched on the horizon of untelling because we simply wouldn't understand.

Guidelines for a new paradigm might be necessary to check ourselves and keep ourselves and our friends on track. From everything we already know, risk would head the list.

RISK. Most persons unfortunately become involved in spirituality or religion not out of a desire to risk, but out of a desire to be made to feel secure in a belief system or worse, a moral code that allows them to subtley judge and be reinforced in that judgement. Movement toward complete integrity of love in body as well as mind and soul will risk misunderstanding and be persecuted by pat judgements. A concept that allows physical love total freedom once a tender context has been established is foreign because it is based on trust of the genuine power of being and nature to find its own truth and resolution. Tender love also does not become a new moral code, i.e. we have all decided that this is good for you, so what is wrong with you if you decide not to participate?

Any posture that pressures and determines what is right and wrong belongs to a sexual category not a tender one. Engendering false security and moral superiority is just one way of being exclusive, not inclusive. The former again, is part of a sexually centered approach, while an inclusive posture opens outward to reverence the freedom, even the freedom to say no, of a beloved.

Shame. It may seem peculiar to mention shame in an age where this emotion has been categorically pummelled as a useless waste and disease. Tyrrell mentions an interesting etymology for the word "shame" as originating from the German

"Scham" and having roots of meaning as "relationship".[cxix]

Though tender touch will eliminate most unhealthy forms of shame, those affecting self image and sexuality, shame in the context of relationship is a valuable guide in negotiating our own tender encounters. The German "Scham dich" or "shame yourself" can be taken in the sense that the person is bad, or it can be a wake up call that the behavior in question is keeping the individual from authentic, loving kinship with another person or group of individuals, or an entire community.

Feelings of shame can be a red flag that physical or emotional overtures disguised as "tender" are more in keeping with the giver's self esteem or ego than reverance for the freedom and divine consciousness of the recipient. Shame can keep us vigilant and self aware, and be a valuable tool in discernment of the spiritually embodied source of our love.

Nonpleasure. Similarly, like shame, this may seem odd. But the desire to please is at the core of the word "pleasure" and this is a sexual and genital posture. I remember attending a workshop once on the ancient form of self discovery called the Enneagram. The group I was in was predominantly church oriented, and the bulk of the individuals present came out to be the number "2" personality type, which are the people server/pleasers. The reason for this disproportionate crowd of "twos" was that people serving/pleasing was intrinsic to many of the staid notions of church as serving, loving others. The downside, however, is the manipulative and exclusive nature of people pleasers.

"This is a kind of clinging to the other and drawing attention to themselves by finding some way to be of personal service. They simply need to be needed. Even without their realizing it, a selfishness creeps into their concern to help. This selfishness desires that the other gives them attention, appreciates them and needs them. A sign that this is so is the way TWOS become quite furious if the other does not take notice of what they have done to please."[cxx]

Since genitally focused actions require the participation of the other, and are a mutual congress of pleasuring, similarly, the desire to please as needing the response of the other, becomes a guide to discovering whether our actions are truly tender or ego centered.

Deep and Lasting Bondedness. My conviction is that we establish institutions of life long commitments such as marriage and religious life because we want to believe in and control a love that lasts forever. Contemporary psychology tells us that this is not so, and is but a fairy tale. But it is in fact true that genuine love does last forever. The quality of lasting is another sign of tender love. And the opposite, the falling apart of a relationship is the sign that tender love was either never present, or that one of the two, or an entire group have become distracted from tender love or the power of Divine/Love's consciousness.

The recent passing of Mother Teresa prompted me to pull an old book about her off of my shelf and give it a perusal for anything which might relate to this work. After marking almost every other page, I was amazed at my own awareness of the tender relationship that this woman was imbued with. During a time when other religious communities, time honored commitments, and nonprofit groups are struggling to stay afloat, I could not help but wonder if at the root, it was not Mother Teresa's devotion to relationship that was the cornerstone to her lasting and prolific success.

"The work is only the expression of the love we have for God. We have to pour our love on someone. And the people are the means of expressing our love for God...

That's just what a Hindu gentleman said: that they and we are doing social work, and the difference between them and us is that they were doing it for something and we were doing it to somebody. This is where the respect and the love and the devotion come in, that we give it and we do it to God, to Christ, and that's why we try to do it as beautifully as possible...There we have Jesus in the appearance of bread. But here in the slums, in the broken body, in the children, we see Christ *and we touch him*."[cxxi] (Italics mine)

Like Jesus in the appearance of bread, we are called to remember. The sufi disciple similarly remembers his master more and more. The bonding which occurs is something deeper than the pleasing or sexual relationship, and is even deeper than the parent and child bond. St. Clare proposed in her rule regarding the infirm, "for if a mother loves and nourishes her daughter according to the flesh, how much more lovingly must a sister love and nourish her sister according to the Spirit!"[cxxii]

Unique. Tender relationships are never boxed away. There are no lovers, or very best friends. Space and time, even great distances (especially in our day and age!) cannot diagram them. Just the selection of "best friend" implies walls and categories that others cannot join, and finally that the "best friend" can betray and break out of.

Tender intimacy may involve sleeping with a friend, literally, just holding one another. It may involve tender lovemaking of an ecstatic and powerful nature. Perhaps it is the shared and natural awareness that you can be comfortable and at peace in your body with another. Each and every relationship, if authentic, must be unique. Otherwise, doing has replaced or is submerging/suspending some or all of the consciousness of love.

Once while in the company of a dear friend, I tried to find a word, or sentiment that seemed to describe each of my close friendships. When I realized that I had yet to find a word for our own relationship. "Oh!" I discovered, somehow regardless of how brave I was being, and how I might be out of place speaking for both of us, "the great wound" I blurted out. Embarrased initially, and not hearing me properly, finally our gazes met as her own recognition settled in.

I watched the woman who had suffered much and shared from that suffering, and supported me in the total freedom gained from her suffering. This same woman had me read out loud the words from Kahlil Gibran, as tears streamed down my cheeks,

"But if you love and must needs have desires, let these be your desires:

To melt and be like a running brook that sings its melody to the night.

To know the pain of too much tenderness.

To be wounded by your own understanding of love;

And to bleed willingly and joyfully.

To wake at dawn with a winged heart and give thanks for another day of loving;

To rest at the noon hour and meditate love's ecstasy;

To return home at eventide with gratitude;

And then to sleep with a prayer for the beloved in your heart and a song of praise upon your lips."[cxxiii]

Then after a long gaze she said the oddest thing, "Now you are ready to write that chapter".

About the Author

The Author brings to the pages of her work direct cultural experiences and relationships with persons at all levels of society, particularly the working poor and single mothers. She owns and operates Miryam Realty, a real estate company which specializes in low-income first-time homebuyers and non-profit agencies. She has taught real estate and has enjoyed past and present memberships in not for profit housing organizations and boards.

Her involvement in human development and spirituality had led her to conduct numerous workshops and lectures over the years, most recently within the Residency Program of the Chaplain's Office at a hospital in Upstate New York.

In addition to writing and research, she is currently a Network Administrator pursuing admission to doctoral studies in Psychology.

[i] Judith Krieger Gardner, ed., *Readings in Developmental Psychology* (Boston: Little, Brown & Company, 1982).

[ii] J. Linn Allen, " Masturbation remains one subject that many won't discuss", *Chicago Tribune*, printed in *Democrat & Chronicle*, (Rochester, New York) 6 February 1995, pg.6,c.

[iii] Janet Sayers, *Sexual Contradictions* (New York: Tavistock Publications, Ltd, 1986), p 75.

[iv] Shere Hite, *The Hite Report* (New York: MacMillan Publishing Company, Inc., 1976), pp 147-150.

[v] Ibid.

[vi] Frederica R. Halligan and John J. Shea, eds, *The Fires of Desire* (New York: The Crossroad Publishing Company, 1992), p 44.

[vii] Halligan and Shea, 72.

[viii] Halligan and Shea, 46.

[ix] William H. Masters, M.D., Virginia E. Johnson and Robert C. Kolodny, M.D., *On Sex and Human Loving* (Boston: Little, Brown & Company Ltd, 1986), 227.

[x] Roger Scruton, *Sexual Desire* (New York: The Free Press, 1986), 120-121.

[xi] Ibid.

[xii] Scruton, 238-239.

[xiii] Halligan and Shea, 112.

[xiv] Gary Smalley, *Hidden Keys to Loving Relationships* (Paoli, PA: Gary Smalley Seminars, Inc., 1993), video series.

[xv] Masters and Johnson,242

[xvi] Masters and Johnson, 243.

[xvii] Scott Peck, *The Road Less Traveled* (New York: Simon & Schuster, 1978), 84.

[xviii] Smalley

[xix] Dr. Joyce Grace and Dr. Mike Grace, *A Joyful Meeting* (St. Paul: National Marriage Encounter, 1980)

[xx] Sheila Kitzinger, *Woman's Experience of Sex* (New York: Putnam, 1983), 240.

[xxi] Llewellyn Vaughan-Lee, *Sufism, The Transformation of the Heart* (Inverness, California: The Golden Sufi Center, 1995), p68.

[xxii] Madelein Gray, "Giving up the Gift: one woman's abortion decision", *Commonweal*, 25 February 1994, p13.

[xxiii] Evelyn Eaton Whitehead and James D. Whitehead, *A Sense of Sexuality* (New York: Doubleday, 1989), 45.

[xxiv] Evelyn Eaton Whitehead and James D. Whitehead, 95,96.

[xxv] Erich Fromm, *The Art of loving* (New York: Harper & Rowe, 1974), 8.

[xxvi] Gay Hendricks, Ph.D. and Kathlyn Hendricks, Ph.D *Conscious Loving: The Journey to Co-Commitment* (New York: Bantam Books, 1990), 144-145.

[xxvii] Paul Pearsall, Ph. D. *Super Marital Sex* (New York: Doubleday, 1987), 198-210.

[xxviii] Anais Salibian, "In touch with yourself, in touch with the world " *Democrat & Chronicle*, Rochester, NY, September 30, 1990.

[xxix] Eustace Chesser, *Salvation Through Sex: The Life and Work of Wilhelm Reich* (New York: William Morrow and Company, Inc., 1973), 28-29.

[xxx] Lisa Ford, *Exceptional Customer Service* video series.

xxxi Lavinia Byrne, ed., *The Hidden Tradition* (New York: The Crossroad Publishing Company, 1991), 34.

xxxii Scott Peck, M.D. *The Road Less Traveled* (New York: Simon & Schuster, Inc., 1978), 84.

xxxiii Thomas Moore, *SoulMates* (New York: HarperCollins Publishers, Inc., 1994), 252.

xxxiv Joan Meyer Anzia, M.D. and Mary G. Durkin, D.Min. *Marital Intimacy* (Chicago: Loyola University Press, 1980), 33.

xxxv Helen Colton, *Touch Therapy* (New York: Kensington Publishing Corp., 1989), 254.

xxxvi Roderick Townley, "Hallelujah! Sex really is good for you!" *Cosmopolitan*, November 1995, 215.

xxxvii Marc David, *Nourishing Wisdom* (New York: Crown Publishers, Inc., 1991), 135.

xxxviii The Classics of Western Spirituality: *Julian of Norwich, Showings* (New York: Paulist Press, 1978), 186.

xxxix Narecia Hamrick, Ph.D. and Grant Bingeman, P.E., *Limitless Intimacy: A Guide to Spiritual Sex* (Dallas: Elysian Press, 1990), 141, 167.

xl Catherine de Hueck Doherty, *Poustinia* (Notre Dame: Ave Maria Press, 1983), 90.

xli Lucinda Lidell, *The Book of Massage* (New York: Simon & Schuster Inc., 1984), 86, 120.

xlii Louis William Meldman, *Mystical Sex* (Tucson: Harbinger House Inc., 1990), 82.

xliii Louis William Meldman, 73.

xliv Robert Calvert, Interview Marion Rosen, *Massage*, Issue number 32, July/August 1991, 49-50.

[xlv] Louis William Meldman, 138.

[xlvi] Gerald G. May, M.D., *Will and Spirit* (New York: The Crossroad Publishing Company, 1986),157-158.

[xlvii] Philip Elmer-Dewitt, "Sex in America", *Time*, October 17, 1994, 64.

[xlviii] Gabrielle Brown, *The New Celibacy* (New York: Ballantine, 1989), 161.

[xlix] Gabrielle Brown, 158.

[l] Daniel Goleman Ph.D., "How to get a grip on anger", *New Woman*, December 1995, 103.

[li] Harvey Jackins, *The Human Side of Human Beings* (Seattle: Rational Island Publishers, 1978), 65.

[lii] Gabrielle Brown, 158-159.

[liii] Narecia Hamrick Ph.D., and Grant Bingeman, P.E., 132.

[liv] John R. Aurelio, *Mosquitoes In Paradise* (New York: The Crossroad Publishing Company, 1985), 37.

[lv] Catherine de Hueck Doherty, *Soul of My Soul* (Notre Dame: Ave Maria Press, 1985), 12.

[lvi] Emilie Griffin, *Clinging* (San Fransisco: Harper & Row, Publishers, 1984), 41.

[lvii] Narecia Hamrick, Ph.D. and Grant Bingeman, P.E., 144-145.

[lviii] Gavin and Yvonne Frost, *Tantric Yoga* (York Beach, Maine: Samuel Weiser, Inc., 1989), 78.

[lix] Gavin and Yvonne Frost, 125.

[lx] Gavin and Yvonne Frost, 79.

[lxi] Stuart Sovatsky, "The Pleasures of Celibacy, "*Yoga Journal*,

March/April 1987, 41.

[lxii] William Johnston *Letters to Contemplatives* (Maryknoll, New York: Orbis Books, 1991), 45-48.

[lxiii] Thomas J. Lyon ed. *This Incomperable Lande* (Boston: Houghton Mifflin Company, 1989), 197.

[lxiv] Ibid, 16.

[lxv] Thomas J. Lyon, 58.

[lxvi] Classics of Western Spirituality *Julian of Norwich Showings* (New York: Paulist Press, 1978), 305.

[lxvii] Jean-Pierre de Caussade *Abandonment to Divine Providence* (Garden City, New York: Image Books, 1975), 25, 26.

[lxviii] Catherine de Hueck Doherty *Doubts, Loneliness, Rejection* (New York: Alba House, 1981), 19.

[lxix] Thomas J. Lyon, 222.

[lxx] Classics of Western Spirituality, 186.

[lxxi] M. Basil Pennington O.C.S.O. *Thomas Merton Brother Monk* (San Francisco: Harper & Row Publishers Inc., 1987), 29.

[lxxii] Jacob Needleman and George Baker, eds. *Gurdjieff* (New York: The Continuum Publishing Company, 1996), 125.

[lxxiii] Frederica R. Halligan and John J. Shea, eds. *The Fires of Desire* (New York: The Crossroad Publishing Company, 1992), 142.

[lxxiv] Benedicta Ward S.L.G. *The Sayings of the Desert Fathers* (Kalamazoo: Cistercian Publications Inc., 1975), 33.

[lxxv] Roger Scruton *Sexual Desire* (New York: The Free Press, 1986), 121.

[lxxvi] John Garvey, ed., *Modern Spirituality: An Anthology* (Springfield: Templegate Publishers, 1985), 75. Karl Rahner's meditation on the Easter Mystery.

[lxxvii] Moshe Idel and Bernard McGinn, eds., *Mystical Union in Judaism, Christianity, and Islam* (New York: The Continuum Publishing Company, 1996), 150.

[lxxviii] Fredrica R. Halligan and John J. Shea, 138.

[lxxix] Jamake Highwater, *The Primal Mind* (New York: Penguin Books USA Inc., 1981), 76.

[lxxx] Tor Norretranders, *The User Illusion: Cutting Consciousness Down to Size* (New York: Penguin Putnam Inc., 1998), 327.

[lxxxi] Hildegard von Bingen, Mensch und Kosmos: Meditationen und Visionen (Guetersloh: Kiefel/Guetersloher Verlagshaus, 1997), 19.

[lxxxii] Coleman Barks with John Moyne trans., *The Essential Rumi* (Edison, New Jersey: Castle Books, 1995), 135,136.

[lxxxiii] Hildegard von Bingen, 34.

[lxxxiv] Op Cit.

[lxxxv] Meister Eckert, *Alles Lassen-Einswerden* (Muenchen: Koesel-Verlag GmbH&Co., 1992), 122.

[lxxxvi] Classics of Western Spirituality, *Meister Eckert: Teacher and Preacher* (Mahwah, New Jersey: Paulist Press, 1986), 243.

[lxxxvii] Classics of Western Spirituality, *Julian of Norwich: Showings*, 319.

[lxxxviii] St. John of the Cross, trans. E. Allison Peers, *Ascent of Mount Carmel* (Garden City, New York: Doubleday & Company Inc., 1958), 308, 309.

[lxxxix] Benedict J. Groeschel, Spiritual Passages: The Psychology of Spiritual Development (New York: The Crossroad Publishing Company, 1986), 188.

[xc] James J. Young, C.S.P., *Growing Through Divorce* (New York: Paulist Press, 1979), p. 9.

[xci] Joann Wolski Conn, ed., *Women's Spirituality: Resources for Christian Development* (Mahwah: Paulist Press, 1986), p. 119.

[xcii] Terence E. Tierney, *Annulment* (New York: Alba House, 1993), p. 51-55.

[xciii] Sam Keen, *A Fire in the Belly* (New York: Bantam Books, 1991), p. 95.

[xciv] James B. Nelson, *Between Two Gardens* (New York: The Pilgrim Press, 1990), p. 51.

[xcv] James B. Nelson, *Body Theology* (Louisville: Westminster/John Knox press, 1992), p. 107.

[xcvi] Stephen R. Covey, *The 7 Habits of Highly Effective People* (New York: Simon & Schuster, 1989), p. 188.

[xcvii] Sheila Kitzinger, *Woman's Experience of Sex* (New York: Penguin Books, 1985), pp. 141 & 138.

[xcviii] Sue Monk Kidd, *The Dance of the Dissident Daughter* (New York: HarperSanFrancisco, 1996), p. 22.

[xcix] Lisa Sowle Cahill, *Women and Sexuality* (Mahwah: Paulist Press, 1992), p. 67.

[c] Rosemary Radford Ruether, *Sexism and God-Talk* (Boston: Beacon Press, 1983), p. 141.

[ci] Elizabeth Johnson, *Women, Earth, and Creator Spirit* (Paulist Press, 1993), p. 68.

[cii] Sandra M. Schneiders, *Beyond Patching* (Paulist Press, 1991), p. 75.

[ciii] Scilla Elworthy, *Power and Sex* (Rockport: Element Books, Inc., 1996), p. 101.

[civ] Jacob Needleman and George Baker, Eds., *Gurdjieff* (New York: Continuum Publishing Company, 1996), p. 33.

[cv] Beatrice Bruteau, *Radical Optimism* (New York: Crossroad

Publishing Company, 1993), p. 112.

[cvi] Narecia Hamrick, Ph.D. and Grant Bingeman, P.E. *Limitless Intimacy: A Guide to Spiritual Sex* (Dallas: Elysian Press, 1990), p. 130-131.

[cvii] Paul Pearsal, *Super Marital Sex* (New York: Doubleday, 1987), p. 210.

[cviii] Jacob Needleman and George Baker, eds. p. 311.

[cix] Gerald G. May, M.D., *Care of Mind/Care of Spirit* (San Francisco: Harper & Row, Publishers, 1982), p. 112-113.

[cx] Carl W. Ernst,Ph.D., Sufism (Boston: Shambhala Publications, Inc., 1997), p. 124.

[cxi] E. Allison Pears,ed., trans., *The Way of Perfection by St. Theresa of Avila* (New York: Image Books, 1964), p. 69, 70-71.

[cxii] Michael H. Crosby. *Celibacy* (Notre Dame, Indiana: Ave Maria Press, 1996), p. 180.

[cxiii] Thomas J. Tyrrell. *Urgent Longings* (Worcester, Massachusetts: Affirmation Books, 1980), p. 51-52.

[cxiv] Sally Cline. *Women, Passion & Celibacy* (New York: Carol Southern Books, 1993), p. 6-7.

[cxv] - Michael H. Crosby, p. 150.

[cxvi] - Subagh Singh Kalsa. *Meditation for Absolutely Everyone* (Boston: Charles E. Tuttle Co. Inc., 1994), p. 66.

[cxvii] Diarmuid O'Murchu, M.S.C. *Religious Life: A Prophetic Vision* (Notre Dame, Indiana: Ave Maria Press, 1991), p. 37.

[cxviii] Francis B. Rothluebber. *Nobody Owns Me* (San Diego: LuraMedia, 1994), p. 87.

[cxix] Thomas J. Tyrrell. p. 103.

[cxx] - Maria Beesing, O.P., Robert J. Nogosek, C.S.C., Patrick H.

O'Leary, S.J. *The Enneagram* (Denville, New Jersey: Dimension Books, Inc., 1984), p. 58.

[cxxi] - Malcolm Muggeridge. *Something Beautiful for God* (Garden City, New York: Harper & Row, Publishers, Inc., 1977), pp. 73 & 87.

[cxxii] Amy Oden, Ed. In Her Words (Nashville: Abingdon Press, 1994), p. 135

[cxxiii] Kahlil Gibran. The Prophet (New York: Alfred A. Knopf, 1983), p. 14-15.